Classics in Psychiatry

ANNALS OF INSANITY

BY WILLIAM PERFECT

ARNO PRESS

A New York Times Company

New York • 1976

616.89
P41
84772

Editorial Supervision: EVE NELSON

—————

Reprint Edition 1976 by Arno Press Inc.

Reprinted from a copy in
  The New York Public Library

CLASSICS IN PSYCHIATRY
ISBN for complete set: 0-405-07410-7
See last pages of this volume for titles.

Manufactured in the United States of America

—————

Library of Congress Cataloging in Publication Data

Perfect, William, d. 1809.
    Annals of insanity.

    (Classics in psychiatry)
    Reprint of the 5th ed. printed for the author,
London.
    1. Psychiatry--Early works to 1900. 2. Mental
illness--Cases, clinical reports, statistics.
I. Title. II. Series. [DNLM: 1. Mental dis-
orders--History. WM P438a 1808a]
RC340.P4 1975   616.8'9'09   75-16726
ISBN 0-405-07449-2

ANNALS OF INSANITY,

Comprifing a Selection of curious and interesting

C A S E S

IN THE DIFFERENT SPECIES OF

L U N A C Y,

MELANCHOLY, OR MADNESS,

WITH THE

MODES OF PRACTICE IN THE MEDICAL AND MORAL TREATMENT, AS ADOPTED IN THE CURE OF EACH.

———⚬✳⚬———

BY WILLIAM PERFECT, M. D.

OF WEST MALLING, IN KENT,

And Member of the London Medical Society.

" *Experto Crede.*"

" *Homines ad deos nulla res proprius accedunt*
" *Quam salutem hominibus dando.*"

FIFTH EDITION.

———◆———

Printed for the Author; and Sold by B. Crosby & Co. Stationer's Court, Ludgate Hill; Messrs. Wilkie and Robinson, Paternoster Row; Mr. Callow, Crown Court, Soho; and may be had of all the other Booksellers in Town and Country.

———◆———

Chalmers, Printer, 13, Castle Street, Leicester Square.

ADVERTISEMENT

TO THE

FIRST EDITION.

By the following cafes, collected with care, chofen with a view to real utility, and reported with precifion and fidelity, it will be eafily feen that the Author has no defign to obtrude any noftrum or fpecific upon the public, but merely to exhibit the refult of his own practice and obfervations in a malady of the greateft importance, in which a confiderable number of perfons are deeply concerned. He has advanced no ideal fpeculations or fantaftic theories, which might furnifh matter of doubtful conjecture, but contenting him-

felf

felf with a faithful recital of facts, unincumbered with tedious and uninterefting particulars, and divefted of ufelefs minutiæ, he trufts that the integrity of his intention will undifguifedly appear to the eye of candour, and ferve to palliate every degree of illiberal criticifm. Be that as it may, of this he is well affured, that fhould the practice of Medicine receive the leaft acceffion from his experience and endeavours, he will think his time well fpent, and his ftudies well directed; and for the indulgent reception of his paft labours the public are entitled to his moft grateful acknowledgments.

DEDICATION

DEDICATION

IN THE

FIRST EDITION.

———

To John Coakley Lettsom,
M. D. F. R. S. ETC. ETC.

Dear Sir,

THE permiſſion which you
have ſo politely granted of dedicating the
following ſheets to you, I regard not
merely as a teſtimony of ſome little pro-
feſſional tenderneſs and ſkill, conſtantly,
however, to the beſt of my abilities exerted towards the relief of ſuch of my
fellow creatures, whoſe complaints involve
the laſt ſtage of human miſery, but as a

proof

proof of private friendſhip, and a record of your own feelings, wherever humanity can be exerciſed or diſplayed. Under theſe impreſſions I will not further treſpaſs upon your time; you will, however, be pleaſed to accept of my moſt fervent gratitude for ſo very reſpectable a ſanction, and permit me to ſubſcribe myſelf,

your moſt obliged

and obedient ſervant,

WILLIAM PERFECT.

ADVER-

ADVERTISEMENT

TO THE

SECOND EDITION.

———————

AS it may juftly be prefumed that the Public have already decided on the utility of this felection, by the rapid fale of the firft impreffion, it cannot fail to afford the Author the moft fenfible fatisfaction to offer a fecond edition, revifed, corrected, and enlarged, as an acquifition to the interefts of humanity, delivered on the authority of extenfive obfervation and practice, as a tribute in the difcharge of his profeffional duties, not unworthy a continued and favourable extenfion of public patronage.

CONTENTS

———◉———

CONTENTS.

CONTENTS.

PREFACE.

IT is an obfervation of the learned **Dr.** Johnfon, that "of the *uncertainty* of our prefent ftate, the moft dreadful and alarming is the uncertain continuance of reafon." Infanity, therefore, being the fevereft of all human calamities, "flefh is heir to," neither pains nor expence fhould be fpared to procure the beft information of that mode of treatment which is moft proper to be purfued on fuch truly trying, critical, and melancholy occafions. A mind, exquifitely fenfible, is too acutely agitated by the conduct of thofe in whom we place the greateft confidence and affection; real or fuppofed injuries frequently deprive us of that invaluable bleffing, our reafon, and leave us the wretched victims to feelings too potent for us to

support

support with that fortitude and philoso-
phy, which the generality of mankind ad-
mire; but which it is impossible for many
of them to practise.

The remote and immediate causes of
this disorder, are in many instances difficult to ascertain ; the arcana are frequently inexplicable, and beyond the reach of
human reason; the definition and arrange-
ment too intricate and perplexed to be
conspicuously enumerated; yet the remote
causes may be allowed to consist of two
kinds, bodily and mental; amongst the
former may be reckoned distension, enlargement, inflammation or irritation of
the membranes and vessels of the brain,
phrenitis, fevers, a morbid state of the
viscera, worms, retention of customary
evacuations, repelled eruptions, gout, &c.
&c. In the latter, various passions, as
fanaticism, joy, grief, hatred, anger, jealousy, pride, ill-requited love, misplaced
confidence,

confidence, defertion of friends at a moment, perhaps, when the balm of friendfhip would have foftened poignant forrow,
and the pointed finger of confcious fuperiority, when the voice of comfort was
earneftly and fanguinely expected; thefe
are trials for the human breaft infinitely
too keen and fevere for tender and deli-
cately fufceptible minds to combat with;
the confequence is, that reafon is hurled
from her throne, and the greateft fkill
is often exerted for a long time in vain
to repair the injury, and wipe away the
fenfe of misfortune. *Extreme fenfibility*
may be deemed a weaknefs; if fo, it is the
moft amiable, the moft pitiable, and moft
to be deplored of any that ever occafioned
mental derangement.

The fymptoms of maniacs are fo totally
different, that fome are not to be reftored
even to the dawnings of reafon, without
long-continued coercion, while in others
nothing

nothing but the moſt lenient meaſures and gentle treatment will accompliſh that ſalutary effect, and reſtore the dementated individual to that glorious luminary of the ſoul, and that emanation of the Deity, REASON.

Humanity has taught the Author of the following pages, to treat all thoſe, who through the ſeverity of their afflictions, have been placed under his care, with the moſt complacent aſſiduity; and whenever he has been obliged to uſe a different plan, it has been with regret and reluctance; notwithſtanding he was convinced of the neceſſity there was to adopt ſuch meaſures. He is no friend to others, nor himſelf, who in caſe of extreme urgency, protracts the cure of his patient, through an overſtrained tenderneſs and delicacy.

Senſible that a candid, cautious, and careful peruſal of this publication, will demonſtrate the efforts of one who has

been

irefied maniac; and, confidering the unfortunate as part of his family, amid a plenitude of practice in the courfe of *fifty years*, the Author has made public this repofitory of Cafes from motives of the pureft philanthropy.

In the medical function it is a moft important attribute " *to feel another's woe,*" and *minifter unto the mind difeafed;* to chace away the care and trouble, that haunts and difturbs the imagination; to apply balm to the pangs that agonize the fenfes, to the nerves that tremble, to the ficknefs of the foul, to fupport the mind under the weight of reafon, tottering to its fall, and bending under the moft erroneous conceptions and ideas of the brain; is a tafk humanely efficient in itfelf, as can never fail to *enfure,* the approval of his fellow creatures *gratefully* exemplified in the prefent addrefs to the public, on announcing another Edition of this Book, which the Author flatters himfelf has not been altogether deftitute of fome merit and utility.

been anxious to live not intirely in vain, but prompt, when the divine light of the foul is extinguifhed, to " minifter to a mind difeafed," has inceffantly ftrove to

" Pluck from the memory a rooted forrow,
" Raze out the written troubles of the brain,
" And with a fweet oblivious antidote
" Cleanfe the ftuffed bofom of that perilous ftuff
" Which weighed upon the heart,"

He prefumes to invite the rational and interefted reader to the perufal of a felection of facts, which may not only in fome meafure afford a clue to medical refearches; but in many inftances ferve as a directory to friends and relations, fufpended between miftaken tendernefs and irrefolution, by which means the difeafe is protracted, and the unfortunate fufferer deprived of the early good effects, which a due fenfe of reftraint in a fituation diftant from home, is generally more productive of, than ill-judged domeftic indulgence in the firft ftages of infanity.

Nume-

Numerous patients who, by the Author means, have been reftored to their famllies, the world, and fociety, have no relapfed, but have continued to enjoy that governing principle, that ineftimable bleffing of the human mind, REASON, in that bright perfection with which they were firft invefted by the beneficence of Providence. Cures, likewife, having been performed under fome of the moft hopelefs and unpromifing appearances, will fhew, that the unfortunate maniac fhould never defpair, fince the goodnefs of our Creator is as unbounded as his power is extenfive.

PREFACE
TO THE
FIFTH EDITION

As nothing human is, or can be perfect, the Author of thefe fheets arrogates no other merit to himfelf, than that which originates in a fervent wifh, to contribute his mite to the fervice of mankind; by faithfully communicating the refult of his practical efforts in *affuaging the mind*, labouring under the moft dreadful malady to which our nature is expofed.

Of the medical character highly diftinguifhed for benevolence and humanity, he may be permitted to afk? Is thy mind richly ftored with fcience?—Thy practice crowned with fuccefs?—and then to fay——

Convince mankind a better fyftem fhine,
Impart it freely or make ufe of mine.

Such practitioner will, I am fure, chearfully fubfcribe to the document given by Lucan, in the following line

" *Non fibi fed toti genitum fe credere.*"
Congenial to the generous and liberal fentiment contained in this excellent quotation, ever wifhing to be a friend to the *poor dif-*

Lately Publifhed,

In two large Volumes, Octavo, Price Twelve Shillings,

THE THIRD EDITION, OF

CASES IN MIDWIFERY,

WITH

REFERENCES, QUOTATIONS, AND REMARKS,

AND AN ENGRAVED PLATE OF AN

HYDROCEPHALOUS CHILD,

Founded on the Correfpondence of the late learned and ingenious

DR. COLIN MACKENZIE.

Sold by the Bookfellers in the Title-page.

Of whom may be had, Quarto,

Price One Shilling,

AN ADDRESS TO THE PUBLIC,

ON THE

SUBJECT OF INSANITY.

By the fame Author.
Embellifhed with an elegant Frontifpiece.

ANNALS

OF

INSANITY.

CASE I.

A Gentleman, aged fifty-eight, of vifage rough, deformed, and unfeatured, and naturally of uncommon filence and referve, was in the beginning of January 1779, committed to my care for infanity. His diforder was attributed to a fudden tranfition in his circumftances, which, from being eafy and comfortable, became exceedingly precarious and embarraffed. The fymptoms of his complaint were violent cephalalgia, an uncommon hatred to particular perfons, a continual noife in his ears, and at intervals either a melancholy depreffion, or a frantic elevation of fpirits.

He

He was of a coſtive habit; his water very high coloured; he paſſed whole nights without ſleep, and was frequently much convulſed; his attention was invariably occupied by one objeȼt, and he would exclaim day and night, That he was ruined! loſt! and undone! Draſtic purges, antimonial vomits, ammoniac draughts, ſegapenum, ſteel, and both kinds of hellebore, had alternately been preſcribed. Iſſues, veneſeȼtion, bliſters, cupping, and cold bathing, had ſucceſſively been tried without effeȼt, or the leaſt viſible alteration for the better. He had, however, never been removed from home to a proper place of retirement, or reſtrained from the converſation of perſons whoſe curious impertinence and frivolous attentions, by inflaming his diſcordant ſenſes, tended only to increaſe his malady.

When he was firſt committed to my care, he appeared extremely impatient of the leaſt contradiȼtion; and the moſt eaſy and gentle diſcourſe would often irritate him into a total miſconſtruȼtion of all that had occurred: I therefore excluded him from all unneceſſary

unneceffary converfation, and from every
kind of intercourfe with his friends and acquaintance, until it was obvious that it
might be permitted without any manifeft
injury or difturbance to my patient.

Could the friends of afflicted maniacs in
general, be made properly fenfible of the
mifchiefs that occur from ufelefs converfation and affecting vifits, they would carefully refrain from both.

The injunctions which I prefcribed
were punctually obferved ; otherwife I
might have met with infurmountable ob-
ftacles in the completion of my curative
plan, which was commenced by paffing a
feton between the fhoulders in the direction of the fpine. My patient was confined to a fequeftered and almoft darkened
apartment. I neither fuffered him to be
interrogated nor replied to, nor did I permit any perfon to vifit him but thofe
whofe immediate bufinefs it was to fupply
his neceffary food, which was light, cooling, and eafy of digeftion ; and his drink
was weak and diluting. His regimen, although frequently directed to be fparing

and

and moderate, had never before been properly attended to: a circumſtance in itſelf exceedingly blameable, and only to be imputed to a miſtaken indulgence. His head was ſhaved, and this frequently repeated; and the warm pediluvium was uſed for twelve nights ſucceſſively, which procured him better reſt than he had before experienced. This induced me to adminiſter two or three purges of the kali tartariſatum in barley water, and afterwards to try the effects of opium, which I began with on the evening of the thirteenth day that he was with me, in the quantity of fifteen drops of the tinct. opii camphorat. in a weak camphorated mixture with nitre. This medicine occaſioned him to ſleep an hour or two at a time, and the following day he always appeared leſs irritable than uſual. The opiate was repeatedly increaſed, until his nights became calm and compoſed, and his days paſſed without that perturbation of ſpirits and derangement of idea, that for ſome time paſt had been too apparently viſible. He now began to diſcourſe conſiſtently, ſeldom breaking out

into

into any frantic rhapſodies or paſſionate expreſſions.

This courſe was invariably perſevered in for upwards of three months, obviating the conſtipating effects of the ſedatives employed, by doſes of the kali tartariſatum, repeated at the intervals of every ſecond or third day. The return of reaſon was now obvious: his imagination gaining ſtrength and accuracy, and his ideas becoming more collected. He now ſaw and ſpoke of things as they really were, and of the primary cauſe of his mental infirmity, with rational coolneſs and reſigned moderation. The ſeton was permitted to diſcharge, but the opium and the pediluvium were gradually decreaſed, and on the ſecond of June following entirely relinquiſhed; when having continued under my care nearly five months, I reſtored him to his friends in that ſtate of ſanity which he has happily preſerved to the preſent time.

CASE

CASE II.

ON the twenty-ninth of September
1770, I was confulted by letter refpecting
the cafe of a gentleman of Carey-ftreet,
London. He was about twenty-two
years of age, and till within twelve months
before had enjoyed a firm undifturbed
mind, with good bodily health. In confe
quence of a matrimonial difappointment,
his difpofition, from being lively and cheerful, became fad, dull, morofe, and penfive,
fubject to watchings, and fond of folitude.
His ufual firmnefs and refolution had entirely forfaken him, and he fuffered under
an almoft entire privation of appetite,
fleep, and fpirits. He was fo dull, dejected, and referved, as fcarcely to fpeak a
word for feveral weeks together; and his
complexion, from being florid and healthy,
became pale and fickly, with a diminifhed
fecretion of urine, feldom voiding more
than a cupful in a day and night. About
three months after this, he was affected
with a ptyalifmus, which continued four or
five

five days without intermiffion; during
which time he difcourfed with his natural
reafon and fluency. His appetite returned, he flept better, and enjoyed a partial
return of his accuftomed fpirits and vivacity; but upon the ceffation of this difcharge, his former gloomy and depreffed
appearance recurred. The ptyalifm returned periodically every full moon, producing its exhilarating, and leaving its defponding effects.

After continuing thus during eight
months, he was entrufted to my management and care on the fifth of January
1771. Finding that many approved and
regular methods of treatment had been in-
effectually adopted, and fuppofing by this
difcharge of the falival glands that Nature
had adopted this mode of relieving herfelf,
and as the patient was not in that ftate of
laxity to prohibit the experiment, and his
friends extremely defirous of trying it, I
refolved to prolong the next periodical
flux of faliva, by the exhibition of calomel
prefcribed at proper intervals, and in
quantities proportioned to his ftrength:
therefore,

therefore, about a week before the expected return of the difcharge, I gave him two
grains of calomel every night at bed-time,
made into a pill with conferve of rofes and
powder of rhubarb. The fifth day after
this his breath became offenfive, and he
complained of a flight forcnefs in his
mouth and gums. On the fixth day in
the evening he began to fpit, which was
moderately encouraged, and the patient
fupported with a regimen fuitable to his
fituation. He appeared focial, cheerful,
and contented, and made no other complaint than that of the tendernefs of his
mouth and gums. I continued to promote the flux in a fmall degree; and as he
was of a weakly habit, the cortex peruvianus was adminiftered twice a day, taking
at intervals an emulfion with neutral falts,
the better to act upon the urinary fecretions, until he had paffed the next full
moon; when obferving that there was no
vifible increafe of the fpitting, I now began to purge off the mercury by lenient
cathartics: but the difcharge did not
entirely ceafe till nearly the end of the
                                        feventh

feventh week from the beginning of the mercurial courfe.   I then opened an iffue in his arm, advifing a cathartic draught, compofed of the kali tartarifatum, with a cool and fparing regimen at the approach and until the decline of every full moon.   The fpitting never after returned, nor was he ever again fubject to thofe mental affections, which ufed to recur at its remiffion.   The cortex peruvianus was for fome time continued to brace and reftore the fyftem, which had been confiderably relaxed and weakened.

Being thoroughly recovered, he left my houfe on the fecond day of May 1771, in a ftate of perfect health and fanity.

CASE III.

MR. S. G. about forty-five years of age, after having been for fome time afflicted with acute rheumatic pains in the joints, and the hæmorrhoides cæcæ, on a fudden, without

without any apparent caufe became ne-
gligent in his drefs, indolent in his manner, low-fpirited, dull, and melancholy,
fo as not to be capable of attending to
his bufinefs as ufual ; he was frequently
watchful, timorous, miftruftful, and defpondent ; and more than once, had he
not been providentially prevented, would
have terminated his exiftence. He was
attacked in the beginning of September,
1772, when he tried the advice of an apothecary who lived near his refidence. On
the November following I received a mef-
fage requiring my attendance, and found
him fitting in his cuftomary penfive and
dejected attitude, his head reclining upon
his arm, with his eyes fixed on the ground
as if loft and abforbed in profound meditation. Several methods were tried to
roufe his attention, but in vain ; I afked
him feveral queftions, but received no
anfwers. I was informed that he had
taken vomits, purges, electuaries, and
mufk. He had a fœtid volatile mixture
to take every fix hours, and a blifter had
been kept open between his fhoulders :

he

he paffed but little water; his ftomach
and bowels were much diftended with
wind; his pulfe was flow, and a flight
hæmorrhage had occurred from the internal hæmorrhoids for fome days, but
had now ceafed.   On the day previous to
my firft vifit he had ejected from his
ftomach a quantity of dark-coloured bile,
with which his ftools were alfo tinged.
Little or no regard had ever been paid to
his regimen, and his appetite was very
indifferent at the beft of times.   He had
been permitted to indulge it with favoury
meat, rich fauces, and other viands that
were calculated to inflame inftead of allay his diforder.   Wine, malt liquor, and
fometimes brandy, had not been denied him; and his unwillingnefs to move
had prevented him from taking that exercife in the open air that might have proved falutary and beneficial.   When I firft
admitted him into my houfe, his afpect
was the moft incurious I ever beheld, and
nearly approached to what characterifes
confirmed idiotifm.   A fervant was obliged to drefs and undrefs him, to give him
his

his food, and in fact to affift him in all the common offices of life.

After a few days I took from him fix ounces of blood, the complexion of which proved the veffels to be loaded with a fuperabundant quantity of humours, that impeded the circulation, fo as to render depletion highly neceffary. I prohibited his wonted freedom of diet, and confined him to abftemious and cooling aliment. He was often carried into the air, and two drachms of the kali tartarifatum were daily adminiftered in a bafon of water gruel. His pulfe was greatly relieved and foftened by the firft bleeding, and by the fecond, at the diftance of fourteen days, the effect was ftill more promifing ; and by a ftrict perfeverance in the antiphlo-giftic plan, repeated bleedings, according to the ftate of his pulfe, with medicines of a ftimulating and antifpafmodic power to increafe the action of the primæ viæ, and a proper degree of exercife, the patient became fufceptible of the dictates of propriety, and regularly attentive to the functions of nature ; and his regimen

was

was gradually enlarged as he recovered his fenfes and underftanding. A fhort time after, valerian and bark were given to invigorate the fyftem, and he left me perfectly reftored to health.

Since effecting this cure, I have had feveral melancholics under my care, who have experienced great relief from the free ufe of the lancet, that in many cafes of this nature appears to have been omitted from an erroneous prejudice. When the pulfe is oppreffed, contracted and hard, and the folids are too much relaxed to affift and increafe the circulating fluids, and promote the fecretions, experience fanctifies the indication, and renders the operation not only juftifiable, but indifpenfible, particularly in more robuft and fanguine habits.

A particular cafe of this nature occurred in the courfe of my practice in this county. My patient was a woman of the name of Cornwall, about four-and-forty years of age, of a plethoric habit, who, had long been immerfed in melancholy. Venefection had been prohibited by thofe

of

of the faculty who were confulted, and yet this patient actually recovered her fenfes by repeated bleedings alone, and has remained perfectly well ever fince.

CASE IV.

A LADY in the thirty-feventh year of her age, of a delicate conftitution, on ly-ing-in with her fecond child, was feized with a fhivering fit that was fucceeded by fever, delirium, and inflammation in the eyes. She was attended by gentlemen of the firft profeffional eminence, by whofe affiftance in the fpace of three weeks fhe was fo much recovered as to be able to walk acrofs her room, when on a fudden, from a miftaken apprehenfion of the fide-lity of her hufband, fhe became reftlefs, anxious, and irrefolute ; turbulent and incoherently talkative ; and fhe was fo very fpiteful and mifchievous that her attendants were obliged to confine her. Spafms, raving, foaming at the mouth, involuntary

involuntary laughter, or loud fhrill lamentations alternately enfued. From a pleafing, open, and cheerful countenance, her
face was contracted into a rigidly emaciated and truly maniacal appearance : and
from a decent and delicate felection of
words, her expreffions degenerated into
the rankeft blafphemy, or difplayed the
fouleft obfcenity. The phyficians that
had attended her, had caufed her to be
bled four times in the fpace of three
months ; blifters had been applied to the
occiput, back, and legs ; a feton had been
made in her neck. To lenient purgatives
brifk cathartics had fucceeded by way of
revulfion ; the foetid gums, and other an-
ti-hyfterics, had proved ufelefs ; vomits,
cupping, and cold-bathing had fucceffively been repeated.

All thefe painful applications, and every
method hitherto adopted had aggravated
rather than extenuated her complaint ;
and in May, 1773, thus fituated, fhe was
configned to my care. She had then an
iffue in her arm, and a blifter on her
back ; but as no fuccefs had followed
from

from mufcular irritation, they were both permitted to heal, and in a few days there was no difcharge from either.

I placed her in a quiet and retired apartment, and gave her occafionally the foda phofphorata, or magnefia, to relax the bowels; ordered the warm pediluvium to be continued every night at bedtime, and a faline mixture with nitre; to which in the evening was added five grains of camphor and a few drops of the tinct. opii. camph. She likewife took mufk in the form of a pill, and made ufe of the warm bath. In a few days the fpafms abated, fhe became lefs impetuous and verbofe, the febrile heat was allayed, and her pulfe, from a hundred and upward, was reduced below eighty. A decoction of peruvian bark, with camphor and nitre, was adminiftered. Her lucid intervals, which at firft continued only a few hours, were in the fpace of a month protracted to a whole day and night; and in a fortnight afterwards to twice that period; gradually increafing until the maniacal fymptoms had entirely fubfided.

During

During her medical courfe, I permitted no perfon to vifit or converfe with her, but my-felf and her female attendant. Her relations and acquaintance were ftrictly enjoined not to difturb her by affecting vifits, which advice and precaution they obferved with the moft punctual attention and deference. Through adhering to this practice and management, I had the fatisfaction of re-ftoring this lady to her worthy partner and family, and to the cordial congratulations of a numerous circle of genteel acquaint-ance, who had experienced much anxiety and folicitude from her deplorable fitua-tion.

CASE V.

A Lady, about forty years of age, from a violent fanatical affection that poffeffed her mind, for fome months became indif-ferent to every enjoyment of life, and was unable to perform the domeftic duties of her family. She had given feveral evi-

c dent

dent proofs of infanity. Her ideas in general were confufed, gloomy, and diftreffed; her apprehenfions without foundation, and her life fo burthenfome, that had fhe not been prevented, fhe would actually have committed fuicide. In this unhappy fituation fhe was conveyed to London for advice, and had feveral vomits and other medicines prefcribed, which are ufually given to patients in a fimilar ftate; particularly the tinct. melampodii, the *fpecific efficacy* of which, as well as the anti-maniacal quality of hellebore, of which the ancients had fo high an opinion, feem founded neither upon truth or experience, as has been particularly evinced in this cafe, and in many others in the courfe of my practice. A blifter had alfo been applied to the back, and ordered to be kept open, but was dried up in much lefs time than it could reafonably be expected to produce any good effect.

Her relations, for the convenience of her being near them, removed her in March 1773, to my houfe. On her features were ftrongly impreffed a pale and
fettled

fettled melancholy ; her eyes looked wild
and ftaring, and her nights were watchful
and reftlefs ; fhe difcourfed on religion in
a ftrange, timorous, defpondent, and incoherent manner, fo that it became abfo-
lotely neceffary to remove from her fight
all books of that nature. When fhe could
procure them, fhe was continually brood-
ing over their contents, to the obvious and.
manifeft increafe of her doubts, fears, and
anxieties. The fervant that attended her,
had orders on no pretence whatever to
fpeak or converfe with her on religious
topics. Her confinement had hitherto
been too clofe, and as air and exercife
were both neceffary for her, fhe was taken
out in a chaife every day. Her pulfe being hard and oppreffed, I foon after fhe
was admitted to my care extracted fix
ounces of blood from her arm, and adminiftered a bolus of nitre every night and
morning, with equal quantities of caftor
and camphor, and occafionally a fmall
dofe of the ol. ricini, to keep the bowels
in a proper ftate of laxity. About the
clofe of the third week the bleeding was

repeated,

repeated, and in a few days afterwards an habitual expectoration that had ceafed from her firft being taken ill, returned, which was affifted by antimonial preparations and the oxymel of fquills; and other falutary ex-cretions following, fhe daily recovered firm-nefs of mind, and renovation of reafon.

At the end of nine weeks fhe returned home, to the great fatisfaction of her family and friends, who have fince cheer-fully confirmed the above cure by the grateful relation of it to their general acquaintance, and confiderably to the credit and advantage of the practitioner.

CASE VI.

ON the fourth of June 1773, I was confulted in the cafe of Mifs L. H. aged twenty-feven, who from an amenorrhæa was afflicted with lownefs of fpirits, vio-lent tumors, hyfteric fuffocation, lofs of appetite, bad digeftion, fpafms, watchful-nefs, palpitation, and diminifhed perfpira-tion.

tion. She became averfe to company and converfation; and when at any time fhe fpoke, it was in a vague, trifling, and whimfical manner, the direct reverfe of her ufual difcourfe; fhe moaned and fighed as if fhe was troubled with the moft grievous affliction. At length, notwithftanding the repeated trials of medical affiftance, by bleeding, cupping, electricity, anti-hyfterical remedies, vomits, neurotics, and emmenagogues, fhe fell into a deep and profound melancholy. Her pulfe, when I firft vifited her, was fmall and irregular, but was rather hard and accelerated; fhe had a conftant throbbing in the temporal artery, and was troubled with a dry convulfive cough. Her urine was pale and limpid, and fhe was frequently affected by the globus hyftericus, with naufea and vomiting.

I prefcribed for her a weak antimonial emetic, and afterwards lac ammoniacum, with fp. nit. dulc. and the oxymel fcillæ; this medicine was continued for three weeks, and finding it did not produce any good effect, another antimonial emetic was administered,

adminiſtered, and ſhe was put under a
courſe of valerian and ſteel, by way of
experiment. This, after ſix weeks, proving
equally inefficacious, and the patient grow-
ing worſe rather than better, on the fifth
of Auguſt I ordered her head to be ſhaved,
and began to uſe the warm pediluvium,
which was continued every evening without intermiſſion.

Two ſcruples of camphor were given her
every day, with fifteen drops of the tinct.
opii camph. in the form of a bolus ; and
although ſhe perſpired freely during the
night, and particularly towards morning,
her pulſe was much quickened, and ſhe
complained of being very thirſty ; for
which reaſon fifteen grains of ſal. nitri
were added to her medicine, which was
taken at bed-time, and at three o'clock in
the morning. The pediluvium was alſo
regularly continued. After each bolus,
ſhe drank a cupful of infuſion of horſe-
radiſh made a little warm, and on the
twenty-fifth of the ſame month ſhe had a
return of the menſtrual diſcharge, which
had been long ſuppreſſed, and in their
ufual

ufual quantity, continuing four days, which was the cuftomary period of their duration.   The tumors abated, the hyfterical fuffocation fubfided, the pains in her head and ftomach were gradually appeafed, her fleep was longer and more refrefhing, and her converfation was rational and uninterrupted.   The boluffes were regularly continued till the fourth return of the catamenia from its firft appearance. Her diet had been particularly attended to during the cure, and principally confifted of nourifhing fpoon-meats and diluting liquids.   As fhe grew better, and the fyftem became re-invigorated, fhe gradually returned to a more folid and liberal regimen; a fmall quantity of wine was mixed with her barley-water, a beverage to which fhe had always fhewn great partiality.   Since this time fhe has continued exceedingly well, and without the leaft return of any maniacal complaint.

CASE

C A S E   VII.

MRS. B. a married lady of about thirty, of a leuco-phlegmatic habit, naturally inclined to melancholy, and of an inert difposition, was in May 1774, from the lofs of a near relation, deeply affected with defpondent ideas. She paffed whole nights and days without uttering one word, and was frequently averfe to receiving any fuftenance : fhe was fubject to loathings, diftenfion of the ftomach, and heart-burn : had frequent inclination to vomit ; would often burft into a flood of tears, and cry with all the vehemence of acute affliction : her countenance was pallid and fwelled, her afpect dejected, and her eyes in continual motion : her urine was fometimes inclined to a red colour, with a lightifh fediment ; and fometimes it emitted fabulous concretions, at others it was generally white and pellucid : her voice was faint, and nearly incapable of diftinct articulation : her tongue was dry, dark, and tremulous ; and her pulfe contracted, hard, and unequal.

Thus

Thus circumftanced, her relations applied to me: fix ounces of blood were taken from her arm, which, when cold, was covered with a thin cake of gluten, that adhered to the fides of the veffel, and fwam in a great quantity of faffron-coloured ferum: foon after the bleeding, fhe took an antimonial emetic, and difcharged a quantity of dark bile.   On the day following fhe began to take two fcruples of camphor every night and morning; on the eighth day of its continuance, an eruption of minute red pimples, refembling the herpes miliaris, in diftinct circles, broke out over all the furface of her body; and the day following fhe menftruated, which fhe had not done before fince the commencement of her derangement; and in a few days after fhe recovered her voice.   The apepfia left her, her countenance partly refumed its natural clearnefs and animation, and fhe began to converfe with her accuftomed propriety.   The camphor was continued, with a fmall addition of nitre, to the thirty-feventh day from its firft exhibition.   At the end of

fix

fix weeks, being as well as fhe had been for many years, fhe was difcharged from my houfe.

CASE VIII.

THE unfortunate man of whom I am about to fpeak, and whofe cafe difplays an inftance fcarcely to be found in the annals of furgery, was game-keeper to a gentleman at Mereworth, a village near this town; he was in the forty-fifth year of his age, and of a tall and flender fta-ture: his countenance was melancholy, his temper gloomy, fullen, and vindictive: having experienced for fome time great difcontent of mind, caufed by an un-expected change in his circumftances, he became dull, filent, morofe, fond of foli-tude, and difturbed in his imagination.

In the evening of the fifth of July 1774, he ftrayed away from home, and not re-turning at his ufual time, the family were greatly alarmed for his fafety: thefe ap-prehenfions were, as appears in the fequel,

but

but too well founded. At midnight he was difcovered by thofe who had been in fearch of him, ftretched on the ground in the hollow of an unfrequented meadow, weltering in his blood, with his throat cut in a moft fhocking manner. The hæmorrhage, which had been very confiderable, being now entirely ftopped, he was capable of informing them that he had perpetrated this rafh and dreadful action himfelf with a razor that he had long carefully concealed for that purpofe. After he was brought home, a furgeon in the neighbourhood was fent for, who reunited the divided parts by future, and attended him daily, but with the greateft defpair of his recovery; and which appeared to every perfon who faw him morally impoffible. On the fixth day after the accident, the ftitches broke loofe and floughed off with the digeftion of the wound: a horrid wound of fix inches in extent now appeared, dividing the fterno hyoideus mufcle, the coraco hyoideus, and the larynx immediately above the thyroid cartilage, and more than two-fifths of the oefophagus.

œfophagus. The air that tranfpired from
the trachea was nearly fufficient to blow
out a lighted candle; but his fpeech and
articulation were not fo much altered and
impeded as might have been expected
from the nature of the wound : confidering its fituation, it is really wonderful how
the carotid arteries and internal jugular
veins efcaped uninjured.

After a confultation of his friends, on
the thirteenth of July, it was agreed to
remove him to my houfe; for which purpofe proper affiftance were fent to his
refidence ; but he fhewed fuch a marked
diflike and reluctance to the meafure, that
notwithftanding his emaciated condition,
and the painful embarraffment of fo dangerous a wound, it was not till after a
ftruggle of nearly half an hour that four
perfons were able to fecure him.   He
was then placed in a chaife, and conveyed
to Malling, when upon a thorough infpection of the wound, and finding the repetition of the futures impracticable, we continued cleanfing and dreffing the parts
twice a day; keeping the head continually
inclined

inclined forwards; by means of bandage the lips of the wound were continued in clofe contact. His food entirely confifted of fpoon meats, in the tranfit of which there was much difficulty of deglutition. At the time of feeding him, unlefs fome refiftance was made from without, very little paffed into the ftomach, but came chiefly through the divided parts upon the dreffings. Yet, aftonifhing as it may feem, in lefs than fix weeks the parts were fo well healed that he could actually and without any great impediment fwallow folids, and the aperture of the wound became fo contracted as fcarce to admit the end of a quill.

At this crifis, from motives of economy, it was judged expedient to remove him to Bethlem Hofpital, where he was admitted in a ftate of bodily health much beyond the expectation of every perfon who had the leaft knowledge of his cafe; and I have fince received authentic information, that the wound is entirely clofed, and the cicatrix perfectly firm, even, and complete; but that he has ever fince continued in

a ftate

a ſtate of inſanity, and been obliged to be cloſely watched and confined to prevent his effecting the act of ſuicide, towards which he ſtill retains an invincible propenſity.

CASE IX.

A Gentleman univerſally reſpected for the integrity of his conduct, having acquired an affluent fortune, at the age of fifty-eight retired from a very proſperous buſineſs, to which he had ever paid the moſt indefatigable attention, to the country, to ſpend a life of uninterrupted eaſe and tranquillity, and enjoy the *otium cum dignitate;* not conſidering that the exertions he had ſo induſtriouſly employed for the attainment of his wealth, were alſo the ſources from which he derived his health and ſpirits; that habit is often more powerful than principle, and that the energies of a mind accuſtomed to an active life, languiſh for want of employment. It is well obſerved by a celebrated divine,
" That

" That when the mind is fuffered to re-
" main in continued inaction, all its powers
" decay, it foon languifhes, and the plea-
" fures which it propofed to obtain from
" reft, end in tedioufnefs and infipidity.
" In this languid, or rather torpid ftate,
" a man has generally fo many vacant
" hours, and is fo much at a lofs to fill up
" his time, that his fpirits utterly decay;
" he becomes burthenfome to himfelf, and
" to every one around him; and drags
" with pain the load of exiftence, weary
" of himfelf and all things about him; his
" fpirits are oppreffed with a deadly gloom;
" and the complaint burfts forth of " odi-
" ous life," and of a miferable exiftence.
" The internal mifery he indures, has
" fometimes arifen to fuch a height, as in
" a dark moment of defpair to make him
" terminate a life which he felt to be in-
" fupportable." And as the following
lines apply ftrictly to the fame fubject, I
fhall here infert them.

" Though each dull plodding thing, to ape the wife,
" Ridiculoufly grave for leifure fighs;
" His boafted wifh from bufy fcenes to run,
" Grant him that leifure—and the fool's undone.
                                    " The

" The gods, to cure poor Damon, heard his vow,
" And bufinefs now no more contracts his brow;
" No real woes, 'tis true, perplex his breaft,
" But thoufand fancied ills his peace moleft;
" The flighteft trifles folid troubles prove,
" And the long ling'ring wheel of life feems fcarce
    to move."

But to refume my narrative. He had
not been longer than four months in the
fituation which he had fo miftakenly de-
picted to himfelf as the completion of his
wifhes, when a liftleffnefs enfued, and he
became fo weary of life as to wifh for its
termination. The corpulency to which
he was naturally difpofed, increafed to fuch
a degree as to render it exceedingly troublefome: he found himfelf depreffed, without being able to define the caufe: he
complained of an uncommon ftricture
about the fcrobiculus cordis; his breaft
became enlarged and fwelled; his appetite
depraved; and his imagination bewildered
with confufed ideas. He complained of
a violent and tumultuous beating of the
carotid arteries, which was perceptible to
the eye: the abdomen was tenfe and coftive: he made but little water, and that
in

in general was thin and colourlefs: he
complained of pain in his head and in his
left hypochondrium, with tenfion and heat
in the parts, and was remarkably thirfty
and feverifh : he was fubjeĉt to cardialgia,
and acid eruĉtations ; impaired fmell,
fpafmodic pantings, and extravagant behaviour ; tremors and dimnefs of fight ;
which terminated in a melancholy delirium. Had he not been carefully watched
and attended in this deplorable fituation,
he muft have fallen by his own hands; he
was fullen and mute, and frequently feized
with a gnafhing and grating of his teeth,
and with involuntary catching of the ten-
dons, yawning and ftretching.

It was with much difficulty that the
phyfician who attended him, could obtain
any kind of anfwer to the neceffary inter-
rogations. This gentleman prefcribed
for him with that judgment and difcern-
ment that had long eftablifhed the reputation of his diftinguifhed medical abilities :
iffues were opened, blifters applied, emetics
adminiftered, and baths made ufe of ; but

in

in vain : he still became worse, even to the heaviest pressure of melancholy.

In this state he was removed from his own house to mine ; his tongue was generally dry, harsh, and discoloured ; his countenance of a sallow hue, dry, and dejected ; his eyes were fierce, staring, and prominent ; the eye-lids constantly tumified, and the pupils uncommonly dilated ; his pulse was full, hard, and oppressed, and did not exceed sixty strokes in a minute. He was averse to food ; and it was with extreme difficulty that he could be prevailed upon to take a sufficient quantity for his sustenance. On the third day after being under my care, I took eight ounces of blood from his arm, the serum of which was charged with bile, and but small in quantity. The crassamentum was streaked with lentor, was tough and grumous. His diet, to which too little attention had been paid when at his own home, was regulated at his new appointment, with an exactness much more to be depended upon. A seton was inserted between his shoulders :

ders : a cooling emulfion of nitre was adminiftered at leaft every eight hours ; and
three drachms of the kali tartarifatum
every other night at bed-time in a little
weak broth, which cooled, relaxed, and
purged him.   On the intermediate nights
a fmall pill, which contained half a grain
of antimon. tartarifat. was adminiftered,
and had the good effect of exciting a gentle diaphorefis, to which from the firft of
his illnefs he had fhewn little or no difpofition.   He paffed more urine, that depofited a copious, light-coloured fediment.
On the feventh morning after the firft
bleeding, the operation was repeated ;
when the complexion of the blood was
much improved, its texture lefs tenacious,
and the ferum was clearer and lefs loaded
with bile.   The pulfe became gradually
fofter, and vibrated about feventy times in
a minute.   He replied with more eafe,
and often with a tolerable degree of ra-
tionality.   He appeared not fo dull and
dejected, and was more eafy and governable. The nitrous mixture, foluble tartar,
and antimonial preparations were refpec-

tively

tively continued at longer intervals, until
the latter end of the nineteenth week;
during which time venefection in proportion to his ftrength had been eight times
repeated, and he was obvioufly amended
in every refpect. His tongue became foft
and moift; his countenance, although
rather pale, became clear and undifor-
dered; and his converfation as rational
and unreferved as it was at any period before his illnefs. At his earneft requeft the
feton was fuffered to dry up.

Near the beginning of the fixth month
from his removal, his return home was
fuggefted to me by himfelf and friends;
to which propofal I acceded, advifing him
to ufe fuch a degree of exercife as fhould
be conducive to his health, and to be more
fparing in his diet than he had been before
the derangement of his intellects.

I have fince had the fatisfaction to hear
that my documents had their due weight;
that by occafionally taking a dofe of the
kali tartarifat. and by a well-regulated
exercife, temperance, and moderation, he
fecures to himfelf the continuance of thofe
most

moft valuable of earthly bleffings, a found
mind and healthful habit of body.

CASE X.

IT was with the moft fenfible degree of
fatisfaction, that, from a melancholy ftate
in which the functions of the mind were
much injured, I was enabled to reftore to
his rational faculty a moft worthy man,
and a valuable member of fociety. He
was in the thirty-ninth year of his age,
had long applied to intenfe ftudy, and had
rigidly denied himfelf thofe relaxations
which are fo effential as a temporal relief
and refrefhment, which a mind fo active as
his required from the immoderate fatigue
which attended intellectual refearches.

The original fymptoms of his complaints were a flatulence of the abdomen,
impaired tafte, forgetfulnefs, anxiety, fugitive palenefs, pain in the cheft, tenfion
in the left hypochondrium, indigeftion,
inquietude, watchfulnefs, a fenfation of
weight

weight in the fpine of the back, and a univerfal laffitude and debility throughout the
whole fyftem. In this fituation he applied to
a furgeon in his neighbourhood, who bled
him three times in the fpace of fix days, and
informed me that the blood which had adhered to the fides of the bafon was black,
heavy, and grumous, feparating but very
little ferum, of a greenifh hue. Soon after the firft bleeding, an emetic was prefcribed, which for fome time he thought
of fervice; but finding his ufual pains and
anxiety return, he defired to have it repeated, a requeft that was immediately
complied with. The next day his complaints returned with redoubled violence;
and, to ufe his own expreffion, he felt
an anxiety and pain affect " his heart."
Extreme difficulty of breathing, rigors and
conftrictions of the external parts, lofs of
recollection, with laffitude and ftupor, and
a violent delirium fucceeded this attack:
his mouth was diftorted, he raved furioufly, was confined, and my advice
thought neceffary.

I found his pulfe full, ftrong, and rapid;

pid; his countenance flufhed and inflated; grinding of his teeth, and his eyes fierce and protuberant. There appeared to be an indifpenfable indication for blood-letting, and that even *ufque ad deliquium animi*, which was accordingly done. The blood appeared nearly in the fame ftate as before defcribed; fomentations were ordered to his feet and legs, and a large blifter was applied between his fhoulders. The night following, an antimonial emetic was ordered, which operated according to expectation. The ftupor was rather leffened; but the pulfe continuing too full and ftrong, ten ounces more of blood were taken from him, which did not appear fo black and grumous as before, and contained more ferum, which was of a better colour. The camphor and nitre were next given in equal quantities, and regularly continued twice a day. For the tenfion in the left fide, a liniment of camphorated oil was recommended to be frequently rubbed in with a warm hand. The blifter was kept open, the bleeding repeated occafionally, and in fourteen

weeks the patient, being completely recovered, returned to his friends, and has
fince continued in good health.

In this cafe it was remarkable, that after
the camphor had been given about a fortnight, an eruption of fmall red fpots appeared pretty generally upon the fkin;
and after continuing a few days, difappeared, recurring in about a fortnight,
with itching, and fome degree of heat.

CASE XI.

A Young lady, whofe cafe I fhall next
relate, was in the twenty-fourth year of
her age; of a very delicate frame, a brifk
and lively difpofition, and of very excellent
powers of mind; but from an irregular
flow of the menfes, became fubject to
hyfteric fits, which at length degenerated
into raving madnefs: her words and actions, from being decent and rational,
became wild, inconfiftent, and extravagant; her anxiety was frequent and extreme;

treme; her appetite was fo much depraved, that fhe would eat paper, cinders,
thread, rags, bits of wall, or any thing that
lay in her way; and fometimes fo unna-
turally voracious, as to fwallow her food
without maflication: her breath was exceedingly offenfive, and her countenance
truly hypocratic. She was reftlefs, hot,
and complained of a pain in her back,
loins, and bowels; with a fenfation of heat
about the region of the ftomach. She
had a dry, frequent, and painful cough,
without the leaft expeƈtoration, with pain
and fwelling in her legs and thighs. Her
blood (as I was informed by the furgeon who
attended her, and who had thought proper
to take away a few ounces on account of
her cough, and to moderate her phrenzy)
was florid, of a loofe confiftence, and did
not in the leaft coagulate in the bafon.
She often continued delirious without intermiffion, or the leaft perfpiration, for
three days and nights together: her lucid intervals feldom exceeded a few
hours, and generally happened about the
middle of the day: her ftools were bilious

ous and fœtid, and her urine concreted, copious, and white. Her flesh was flaccid and dry. She would frequently burst into immoderate fits of laughter, which by a sudden transition, turned to involuntary tears; to which succeeded screams, yells, and horrid ravings: her pulse was hard, quick, and small; and she was often seized with fugitive spasms in her hands, arms, legs, and thighs.

On the first of June 1775, she was placed under my care. I commenced the cure with an antimonial emetic, in the operation of which she ejected a very long and broad worm, of that species called the tænia. The warm pediluvium was the same evening made use of, with a course of camphor and nitre, and occasionally a mixture containing castor and musk in equal quantities, with oxymel of squills in pennyroyal water, which was uniformly continued to the end of the cure, with a vermifuge powder of rhubarb and calomel, which I thought proper to prescribe every fifth or sixth night.

During

During more than three months fhe
had fhewn no figns of menftruation ; the
firft return of it was obferved on the 26th
of June, and the 24th of the following
month it returned in a more copious quantity. A few days fucceeding, there was a vifible change for the better. Her mind appeared lefs difturbed and confufed ; the
fymptoms gradually abated, fhe recovered
her mental powers, and has been very regular in her menftruation ever fince, though
at intervals not quite fo rational as before.   While under cure, an eruption,
fimilar to the urticaria, appeared every
fecond or third day on the face, arms, legs,
and breaft ; and at thofe times fhe was
obferved to be moft calm and collected,
and leaft fubject to heat and pain.

CASE XII.

THE patient who is the fubject of this
cafe, had long been afflicted with a com-
plication of complaints, from neglect at
that

that period of life to which the fex in general pay too little attention. She was naturally of a fpare, thin, and relaxed habit; was lame of the right hip, from a luxation of that joint in infancy; and had been accuftomed to copious difcharges of the menftrual flux, a total ceffation of which took place in the thirty-ninth year of her age; foon after which fhe was attacked with an inflammation in her eyes, hæmoptoe, and a pain in her loins, which was tranflated to her head. Thefe were attended with a numbnefs in the hands, finging in the ears, and borborygmi. Her feet and ankles fwelled; fhe was fubject to fpafmodic affections in various parts of her body; to jaundice; a fixed rednefs in both her cheeks, and great inequality of fpirits. By a proper courfe of medicine fhe recovered from moft of her complaints, except the jaundice, which ftill remained, with great indolence and laffitude of her whole body, anxiety, dyfpnæa, and coftivenefs; fhe had a great depreffion of fpirits, frequent ficknefs, and heavy fighings.

The

The lofs of a near relation, who had died in May 1774, fo increafed her affliction, as to render it abfolutely neceffary that fhe fhould be removed from her own habitation to a fuitable recefs for perfons whofe mental derangement caufes fuch a meafure to be indifpenfable. In this fituation her diforder increafed, inftead of abated. When the time expired that her friends had engaged that fhe fhould be there, they thought proper to fend her to me. She feemed much emaciated with grief and vexation, and laboured under the ufual concomitants of melancholy. Her countenance was bloated and yellow, her appetite depraved, her eye-lids tumid and inflamed, the pupils uncommonly dilated, and her whole fyftem diftempered and relaxed. It was in the December following that fhe was placed under my care; foon after which an antimonial emetic was adminiftered, which evacuated a great quantity of bile from her ftomach, with which it had been long loaded: every third night at bed-time a ftomachic purgative was prefcribed, and a mixture

of

of camphor with powder of fquills: an
iffue as opened above her knee.   After
a fortnight the vomit was repeated, and
the morbid contents of the ftomach were
much lefs in quantity than before.   The
ftrength of the patient was increafed by a
light nutritious and diluting diet; but the
camphorated mixture with fquills creating
a naufea, the following form of pills was
fubftituted:

> R Extract Chamom. ʒij.
>   Pulv. Rhei   ℈ij.
>   —— R. Columb. ℈ij. gr. v.
>   Ol. Eff. Carui   gr. iv.
>   Syr. Croci. q. f.   M. f. Pil. mediocr. mag.

Of which fhe took four twice a day, and
continued them during fix weeks, when
fhe was fuddenly feized with a violent
fhivering and reaching to vomit, till the
zona ignea, or fhingles, appeared round
her waift, which being removed by the
antiphlogiftic plan, the menftrual difcharge
returned; and being confiderably better,
fhe returned home, and has ever fince retained a tolerably good ftate of health,
uninterrupted

uninterrupted by any mental infirmity of long continuance.

CASE XIII.

M ISS A. C. of a delicate habit, was subject to nervous affections and painful menftruations. Having for fome time, without any apparent caufe, fhewn evident figns of infanity, fhe was in the month of March 1776, placed under my care. She was naturally of a lively active difpofition, and remarkable for quicknefs of parts. Under the influence of her delirium, fhe fhewed great vivacity of mind, and would often exprefs herfelf in welladapted and really very harmonious meafure ; though when in her right fenfes fhe was never known to have any particular penchant for poetry. She was in continual motion, as if fhe had been bitten by a tarantula, and was inceffantly pouring forth a rapid fucceffion of ideas, which fhe uttered with amazing and incredible facility ;

facility; feldom, either by day or night, giving any reft to her fpontaneous and luxuriant fancy. She was habitually coftive, and particularly fo about the return of her menftrual periods. She had long been much relaxed; and bracing, corroborating, and ftomachic medicines, had been ineffeftually prefcibed. I had therefore recourfe to the auftere and aftringent vegetables. The oleum ricini was occafionally given to remove her coftivenefs, and which fucceeded much better than any other laxative prefcription that had been adminiftered. Its fuccefs in this inftance is to be attributed to the fmall degree of naufea it caufes in the ftomach, and the fhort time it has to irritate in paffing through the inteftinal canal. From the commencement to the end of her menftruation, twenty drops of tinft. opii camph. were given every night and morning in a diluted camphorated mixture, from the fourth of April to the thirteenth of July following. On the feventh of Auguft fhe was difmiffed from my houfe at the defire of her friends, and care having
been

been taken to alleviate the pain occafioned by the menftrual flux, by the foothing influence of fedatives, has, I am informed, remained ever fince free from any return of infanity.

In Van Swieten's Commentaries we are informed of a woman who had feveral times been maniacal, and who in the paroxyfms of infanity always fpoke in metre, and fhewed a wonderful facility at verfification, though at other times, when in her right fenfes, fhe never fhewed any fkill or tafte for any thing of the kind, having been from her youth accuftomed to earn her bread by the labour of her hands, and was not at all remarkable for the quicknefs of her parts.

CASE XIV.

THAT a depravity in the habitual fyftem of the mind will occafion a derangement of its ideas, even to madnefs itfelf, is a fact of fuch notoriety, that a very flight

acquaint-

acquaintance with thofe who labour under mental infirmities, will fufficiently evince its truth: and it may be juftly obferved, that pride is the moft dangerous enemy of mankind, and the fource of innumerable evils. From an habitual indulgence in this deftruƋive vice, I fhall relate an inftance, which although it comes not into my curative point of confideration, having baffled every medical effort of relief, not only confirms the appropriate juftice of this obfervation, but alfo ferves as an introduction to a curious cafe, that I have been favoured with by a correfpondent, who, I believe, fhortly afterwards made it known through the channel of fome periodical print.

The patient was a middle-aged man, not tall, but upright in ftature, remarkable for acrimony in his fpeech and anfwers, impetuofity in his manner, and aufterity in his aƋions. His countenance bore evident traits of pride, fufpicion, and morofenefs; he was naturally of a reftlefs, contentious, and irritable difpofition. From an unexpeƋed mifcarriage in his commercial

mercial affairs, he became intolerably dif-
contented, jealous, rude, difrefpectful to
his family, contemptuous, intemperately
paffionate, and mifanthropic to the greateft
degree.   In this manner his infanity commenced.   He drew upon his banker for
fums immenfely beyond what his accounts
would afford, and when difappointed in
this refpect, became fullen, and immediately iffued drafts upon houfes with which
he never had the leaft connexion, for enormous fums.

Thefe and innumerable other actions
equally *outrè*, fixed the criterion of his
infanity, and determined his relations to
take out a ftatute of lunacy, and to fix
him in a place appropriate to his difordered imagination.   He iffued his man-
dates and decrees with all the arrogance
and felf-importance of an eaftern defpot.
He would often draw upon the bank for
ten or twenty thoufand pounds, with all
that fettled pomp and gravity which
feemed to mark the reality of the tranfaction.   He frequently infifted upon his
being the lord chancellor, king of Spain,

duke of Batavia, or fome other great per-
fonage, and accordingly demanded reve-
rence and refpeƈt ; which homage, if not
paid him, he would immediately become
furly and outrageous, and with great vociferation would give out his orders for
the punifhment of thofe delinquents who
appeared to have been remifs in their
duty and obedience; and would remain
apparently fatisfied, as if he thought his
commands had been punƈtually attended
to. He feldom exprefled the fenfe of any
bodily pain ; nor was bleeding, bliftering,
vomiting, or any evacuations of the leaft
fervice : he was uniformly vain, formal,
and ftately; arrogant, gloomy, and felf-
fufficient ; and however ridiculous his
words and aƈtions appeared to others,
they were fupported in himfelf with all
the dignity of exceffive pride and oftenta-
tion, and a uniform exhibition of that
fpecies of infanity with which he was affeƈted. His imaginary greatnefs and felf-
confequence dwindled into a total decay,
as he approached the verge of idiotifm, in
which abyfs I fhall leave him, to take a
view

view of the communication referred to at the commencement of the cafe. Its analogy entitles it to a place here, as no unfuitable appendix.

The writer premifes the relation, by obferving, that in the long catalogue of infirmities to which human nature is fubject, no one is more terrible than madnefs or infanity. To be deprived of the quality which enables mankind to regulate their conduct, and the defire for their own prefervation, reduces them below a level with the brute creation. This calamity, however, appears more terrible to the fpectator than it really is; for he judges of the feelings of the unfortunate by his own, conceiving what himfelf, endowed with reafon, would experience, if in his fituation. By indulging an idea of what is impoffible, and connecting reafon with infanity, he feels intenfely for the miferable fituation of the lunatic, whilft the latter is infenfible to any other uneafinefs than what arifes from the difappointment of his fchemes, and the burfting of thofe airy bubbles that are formed by his own

heated

heated imagination. In some instances of insanity, there is such an assemblage of sense and madness, that the beholder is compelled to smile as well as compassionate: but the tear of pity will not flow less sincerely down the cheek of sensibility, because alternately blended with involuntary laughter. The following story is added as a proof of this assertion.

Some years ago a poor man, who had studied the art of government and the balance of European power, with greater attention than his business, became insane, and fancied himself a king: in this situation he was admitted into the workhouse of Saint Giles in the Fields, where there then happened to be an idiot of nearly his own age. The imaginary monarch appointed him his prime minister; besides which he officiated as his barber and menial servant, he brought their common food, and stood behind his majesty while he dined, till he had permission to make his own repast. There you might behold the king upon an eminence, and his prime minister below him, for a whole day together, issuing their

precepts

precepts to their imaginary fubjects. In this manner they lived about fix years, when unfortunately the minifter, impelled by hunger, fo far deviated from his allegiance, as to eat his breakfaft before his fovereign. This fo exafperated the king, that he flew upon him, and would have put a period to his exiftence, had he not been fortunately prevented. When his anger was thought to have been appeafed, he was again introduced to his quondam fovereign; but he feized him immediately, and could never be prevailed upon to fee him again. The degraded minifter caught a fever in his exile, and when his majefty was beginning to relent, and was almoft perfuaded to fee him, he died; which had fuch an effect upon the fancied king, that after having lived almoft without fuftenance, in a continued filence, he actually died of grief. Ill-fated monarch! Thou canft not, as the illuftrious fovereign of the prefent day, if his minifter were to pay his tribute into the treafury, to which we muft all be taxed, appoint another who would act with as much prudence and

fuccefs

fuccefs as the prefent one had done.
Throughout the whole territory there was
not one found hardy enough to engage in
the arduous tafk, and equally unable to
fupport the weight of government alone,
as to defcend to the peaceable but unho-
noured vale of retirement. Thou didft
quietly refign thy life and fceptre together.
Perhaps it may be fome fatisfaction to
the reader, to be informed, that this anecdote is founded in fact, his name having
ftood in the books of the parifh, with the
addition of The Lunatic King, for feveral
years. The firft entry being January 1ft,
1727.

Something of a fimilar inftance of infanity
occurs in Wier de Præftig. Dæmon. lib. 13.
de Lamiis. cap. 7. f. 2. Operum, pag. 180.
and may be tranflated in Englifh, as follows. I knew an Italian troubled with
melancholy, who believed he was a monarch, and emperor of the world, and that
he alone had a right to that appellation.
In other refpects he was rational and elo-
quent, and did not labour under any difeafe. He was wonderfully amufed in
compofing

compofing verfes in Italian, relative to the ftate of Chriftianity, and to the putting an end to the war that then exifted between France and Holland, all which he believed to be fo many divine oracles. He every where made known his titles by means of thefe letters, **R. R. D. D. M. M.** or Rex Regium, Dominus Dominantium, Monarchus Mundi; i. e. King of Kings, Lord of Lords, and Monarch of the World. And Cælus Aurelius, in his firft book of Chronic Diforders, chapter 5, page 328, fpeaking of madnefs, fays thus: " One in his raving has fancied himfelf a God, another a tragedian, another a comedian, and another carrying a ftraw in his hand, has imagined that he held the fceptre of the world."

Another inftance of arrogant infanity we find in the following paragraph from a public print. Lately died in the workhoufe in Durham, aged eighty-five, Thomas French, well known in that city for the laft fix or feven years, by the fictitious title of Duke of Baublefhire, which in the diction of his underftanding he affumed

without

without royal creation, and wherein he
feemed to have greater pride than any
peer of the realm adorned with a real
one. He wore a ftar compofed of cloth
of various colours, or of painted paper,
upon his breaft, a cockade in his hat, and
feveral brafs curtain rings upon his fingers. He was fo enthufiaftically enrap-
tured with his vifionary dignity, as to imagine he had frequent conferences with the
king on the fubject of raifing men, carrying on the war, and other important
matters of ftate; in which, however, he
was not more abfurd than many other
infane felf-taught politicians of the prefent day.

CASE XV.

A. N. aged thirty-one, of a bilious and
plethoric habit, from great uneafinefs and
agitation of mind, became infane; many
extravagant ideas entered into her mind,
fhe raved almoft inceffantly, with fhort, but

not

not lucid intervals; fhe would frequently
pray, fhout, laugh, jump, dance, fcream,
and weep; and paid little or no attention
to the exterior objects around her; fhe had
menftruated in fmaller quantities than ufual
for fome time before. Her countenance was
florid, her features were diftorted, her eyes
protuberant, brilliant, and conftantly moving; their lids confiderably tumefied and
inflamed, and the pupils much expanded;
her voice was harfh, hoarfe, and hollow;
fhe had great and extreme heat; her pulfe
was hard, ftrong, and violent, under which
indications the lancet was ufed freely, and
repeated five times in the fpace of as many
days; in which time fhe loft feventy
ounces of blood: between the operations
antimonial emetics were adminiftered, and
a draught with the kali tartarifat. in the
quantity of half an ounce.

Notwithftanding the fmall quantity of
nourifhment which fhe had taken for ten
days paft, and repeated venefection, the
pulfe continued very ftrong and full; and
her bodily ftrength was incredible, without the leaft mitigation of her infane
fymptoms.

fymptoms. Her blood had uniformly
from the firft appeared of too denfe a
confiftence, and when cold, refembled
melted fuet ; nor was this appearance
much more leffened in the laft than in the
firft operation; fo that any correction of the
vicious ftate of the humours was but little
to be expected from bleeding, however that
depletion of the veffels had prepared the
way for the effect of attenuants. Lenient
purgatives, with foluble tartar, were at ftated times repeatedly adminiftered; a feton
was opened between the fhoulders in the direction of the fpine; the camphorated mixture was given two or three times a day ;
and every morning and night fhe took the
extract of chamomile flowers, myrrh, and
fteel, in the form of a pill, with a decoction of horfe-radifh after each dofe; which
method fhe purfued fix weeks, when fhe
began to have lucid intervals of three,
four, or five hours in the courfe of the
twenty-four. Thefe intermiffions, with a
continued ftrict obfervance to medicine
and diet, were gradually prolonged till
they became fo permanent, that at the
end

end of four months fhe was capable of returning to fervice; and has continued well ever fince. She is fince married, and become the mother of a large family.

CASE XVI.

THE fon of a worthy and refpeƈtable magiftrate in the city of London, had, in the feventeenth year of his age, fuddenly, and without any previous fymptoms, been feized with a fpafmodic complaint in his right arm, leg, and jaw, with remitting pains on that fide of the thorax ; and his eyes were red and inflamed, and affeƈted with vifcid defluxions; which fymptoms continued for fix weeks without his experiencing any relief from blifters, finapifms, eleƈtricity, or antifpafmodic medicines of various kinds. About the end of the feventh week from the beginning of the attack, for fome days together the contraƈtions and pain appeared lefs violent; and as the fainteft ray of hope was received

ceived with the moſt ſanguine expeĉtation,
by a fond and indulgent parent, ſo in a
few days when thoſe ſymptoms recurred,
attended with a partial paralyſis of the
tongue, that at firſt rendered the voice
indiſtinĉt, and afterwards entirely incapable of articulation, his paternal feelings
were rendered more intenſe than before.
Thus ſituated, the moſt approved medicines were adminiſtered, and the beſt advice and aſſiſtance given that could then
be obtained ; but to ſo little effeĉt, that at
the end of ſeventeen weeks no alteration
for the better was obſervable : he could
neither read, write, nor ſpeak, ſo as to be
underſtood ; and with difficulty received
his food from the hand of an aſſiſtant.

In September 1775, I received a well-
written letter, deſcribing the caſe with the
greateſt preciſion, and ſoliciting my advice
and opinion.   In my anſwer I expreſſed
my diffidence of rendering him any ſervice, but obſerved, as I had been conſulted, if his removal was praĉticable, and
conſiſtent with the inclination of his
relations, I ſhould rather chuſe to have
him

him placed under my own immediate care, than prescribe for him at a distance. This proposal was readily acceded to, and on the twenty-fifth of the same month he was sent to me. He appeared to be naturally of an extenuated form and make, was much reduced by his illness, and looked pale and wan, with a yellow cast in his countenance. He was now totally deprived of speech; and in walking, which he was scarcely able to do, would suddenly stop, and keep his eyes fixed upon the ground, or some particular object, and continue to stare at it for a considerable time together; and when he took his eyes off, remained sheepish and hung his head, drivelling like an idiot; at times he was slightly convulsed, with costiveness and nausea. His intellects were so much impaired, that he acted in a most indecorous and childish manner. A blister, which for many weeks had been kept open in the back, was now suffered to dry up; an antimonial emetic was administered on the second day after his removal; and a seton was passed between the shoulders,

ders, in the direction of the fpine. On
the fixth, the joints of both arms being
much enlarged and tumefied, leeches were
applied to them, and afterwards warm attenuating cataplafms; embrocating them
with a faponaceous volatile liniment, containing a drachm of tinct. cantharid. until
the tumefactions had entirely fubfided.
The vinum aloeticum alkalizatum, warm-
ed with the tinct. lavendul. comp. was occafionally given to keep the body properly
open; and a diluted camphorated mixture, with antimony and nitre, three times
a day, when the ftomach was moft empty.
The feton difcharged exceedingly well;
and by a ftrict attention to his diet, in lefs
than two months he fo far recovered his
mufcular ftrength, as to be able to walk
about and divert himfelf by playing upon
the violin, which before his illnefs had
been his favourite amufement.   He now
daily became more active, lively, and gay;
and in a little time after was able to write
and hold a tolerably confiftent correfpondence with his friends : and being thoroughly recovered at the end of fix
months,

months, he returned home, has continued free from any bodily complaint, and is now capable of carrying on an extenſive buſineſs, (to which he has ſince become a partner) with the ſtricteſt order, regularity, and attention.

―――――――――

CASE XVII.

A Young man, naturally of a robuſt and ſanguine conſtitution, yet of feeble intellectual faculties, after drinking to exceſs, had his body covered with phlogiſtic blotches, with general fever, a hard pulſe, and topical pains. Falling into unſkilful hands, the inflammation was repelled, and in all probability was the occaſion of ſome tranſlation to the brain. The patient became dull, heavy, and penſive. He had an obtuſe pain in the cheſt, with ſwelling and tenſion in the region of the heart, for which he was bliſtered, loſt blood, and took ſome purgative medicines ; but found no relief: he had reſtleſs nights, and was ſubject to

F   rigors,

rigors, with laffitude and ftupor; was now but little feverifh, and had given many inftances of being infane.

On the eleventh of May 1777, he was entrufted to my care. He appeared to be under much anxiety; his afpect was wild, his countenance florid; a rednefs and inflammation in the tunica albuginea, a white tongue, and difficult deglutition. He complained of the head-ach, was hot, and had but little appetite: his pulfe was hard, ftrong, and above the natural ftandard; and he was fo coftive, that he had no evacuation by ftool for feveral days together. Thefe fymptoms were accompanied by great agitation of mind, and a frantic manner of behaviour; a wild incoherent converfation, hurry, buftle, and uncommon ftrength and reftleffnefs. The indication of inflammatory difeafe being thus evident, venefection was ufed; and the difcharge of twenty ounces of blood not being fufficient to bring on a deliquium, the quantity was increafed to nearly thirty, which fully effected that purpofe. The complexion of the blood afforded little

little or no information; an antimonial
emetic was adminiftered the day after the
operation, and was repeated five or fix
days after at three different times, alternately with the following draught:

> R Kali Tartar.   ʒiij.
>   Mannæ   ʒfs.
>   Aq. Cinnam.   ʒifs.
>   Decoct. Hord. ʒij M. f. Hauft.

But although by this treatment the bodily fymptoms were much relieved, and the
pulfe confiderably lowered, the functions
of the mind were yet much impaired, and
he continued in a kind of torpid ftate
nearly to the end of four months, when
after the free ufe of the warm bath and
camphorated mixture, he fhewed evident
fymptoms of amendment, began to recover
the ufe of his reafon, and for many days
together there were hopes of its continuance. But a relapfe following, and the
maniacal fymptoms recurring in a more
confiderable degree than before, it was
not until a month afterwards that a fecond
lucid interval took place, and he became

fufficiently

sufficiently recovered to go out by himself, and was allowed to walk and derive
benefit from the frefh air and exercife.
Soon after this a profufe eruption, fomewhat refembling the fcabies, fuddenly
broke out on his hands, arms, neck, and
breaft, which was effectually cured by an
attenuating cooling regimen, with laxative
medicines. From this period he continued
to recover without any farther relapfe,
until he was able to return home and purfue his cuftomary occupation.

CASE XVIII.

MARY, the wife of John Ingram, of
Chepftead, in this county, had the misfortune to catch cold during her lying-in of
her firft child, which caufed extraordinary commotion both of mind and body,
and terminated in actual infanity. She
was furious, reftlefs, turbulent, irafcible,
and raved inceffantly : her body was coftive ; her eyes were vivid, diftorted, and
inflamed;

inflamed; her tongue was rough and parched, without thirſt; her ſkin hot and harſh; and her countenance ſallow and bloated: it was with much difficulty that ſhe was reſtrained from doing miſchief to herſelf and others; and after continuing ſome weeks in this ſituation, it was concluded by her friends to conſult me.

On inquiry I found that the lochia, during the period of their evacuation, had been much leſs than uſual; and had totally ſtopped from the time of her being taken in the above manner: ſhe had ſecreted but little milk, and had no perſpiration. Some medical aſſiſtance had been ineffeċtually adminiſtered; and being in ſlender circumſtances, and incapable of preventing it, ſhe had been too much expoſed to idle curioſity, which the vulgar too often are diſpoſed to exerciſe on theſe unhappy occaſions, to the extreme aggravation of the delirious ſufferer; and to the ſhame of every tender feeling and emotion of humanity. As her circumſtances would not admit of removal, perſonal coercion was the firſt thing direċted,

under

under the care of a proper attendant, with a ftrict injunction that all unneceffary vifitors fhould be entirely excluded from the fight of her. A proper quantity of blood being taken away, the texture of which was fizy, and the ferum yellow and turbid, the following emulfion was pre-fcribed :

    R Emulf. Amygd. ℔j.
      Mannæ   ℥j.
      Kali Tart.   ℈iij.
      Sp. Nitri dulc. ℈ij. f. M.
Cyathum exhibend. fecunda vel tertia quaque hora donec fatis purgaverit.

A feton was paffed between the fhoulders in the direction of the fpine, that in a few days began to afford a copious difcharge. As the emulfion was not fufficiently ftrong to effect the defired purpofe, fix drachms of the kali tartar. with an additional quan-tity of manna diffolved in the decoct. hordeatum, was adminiftered every third day for fix weeks fucceffively, and the following drops and mixture on the in-termediate days

                        R Sp.

R Sp. Volat. Fœtid.

Tinct. Lavend. Comp. āā ʒvj. f. Guttæ.

Sumat Gutt. lxx ter in die vacuo Stomachio ex Cyatho Mifturæ fequent.

R Camphor.   ƺiifs.

Sacchar Alb.   ʒvj.

Aceti calefact. ʒxij. M. f. Mift. f. a.

A flender and fpare regimen, and a total abftinence from animal food, was advifed, and plenty of diluting liquids were allowed. In ten days the poor woman became more calm and rational, and obtained fome refrefhing reft at night, that was accompanied with a gentle perfpiration. In fix weeks the cinchona being found neceffary as a tonic, completed the cure.

It is rather remarkable, that the menfes did not return till three months after her recovery, although previous to this illnefs fhe had been exceedingly regular in that refpect. When that period returned, fhe was for fome time troubled with nervous affections, that by the affiftance of the cinchona and valerian were foon fubdued, and her health and underftanding perfectly reftored.

CASE

CASE XIX.

THE ſubjeƈt of the following recital
was a poor woman in the thirty-fifth year
of her age. She had borne three children, and in her lying-in of the laſt, from
ſome improper treatment, was rigorouſly
attacked by ſickneſs and vomiting, and
complained of acute pain in her head and
the region of the womb, with a great degree of tumour, heat, and tenſion. She had
taken a vomit, fomentations had been applied to the abdomen, and other means
had been uſed; notwithſtanding which,
her complaint continued ſo as to af-
feƈt her intelleƈts. After this, ſhe received no farther medical aſſiſtance, and
remained for ſome time tolerably well,
when the pain, tenſion, and vomiting ſuddenly recurred; and ſhe became poſſeſſed
of diſeaſed perceptions, notions, ſuſpicions,
and apprehenſions, attended with vociferations and ſlight ravings; in which ſituation ſhe was conſigned to my care.

Evacuations by ſtool, and antiphlogiſtic
medicines,

medicines, were adminiftered without effect; the pediluvium and emetics fucceeded. From thefe fhe experienced confiderable relief; but although the ftomach
was foul, and fhe ejected a confiderable
quantity of bile, the pain in her head was
much increafed by its operation. Her
diet was regulated according to the indications of the cafe; a blifter was kept
open between the fhoulders; her head
was fhaved; and the acetated camphor
mixture, and common emulfion, with the
fœtid volatiles, were prefcribed to her
three times a day, when the ftomach was
moft empty, and every night at bed-time;
the good effects of which were particularly
apparent, the maniacal fymptoms gradually abated, and in the fpace of two months
the patient was recovered in every refpect,
except a nervous weaknefs, for which the
ufual remedies were exhibited. She was
now difmiffed from my houfe, has remained in better health than fhe enjoyed
for fome time before, and has never
fince had any return of the diforder.

CASE

CASE XX.

H. G. a native of Folkſtone, in Kent, had, from the total ceſſation of the menſes, which occurred ſoon after her forty-fifth year, been much affected in her ſenſes. She was rather of a ſanguine habit, had lived freely, and been accuſtomed to copious evacuations. The menſes ceaſed very ſuddenly, and ſhe ſuffered much from plenitude; for beſides the derangement of her intellects by their ceſſation, ſhe was attacked with the hæmorrhoids, and was coſtive; had fugitive ſpaſms in her arms and legs; a deafneſs, with a ſenſe of weight in the fore part of the head; frequently an obſtructed deglutition; and a univerſal eryſipelas, attended with acute fever, and great heat and pain about the præcordia. It was ſeveral weeks before ſhe was conſidered out of danger.

About twelve months after her recovery from this illneſs, without any apparent cauſe, and after a ſlight head-ach, ſhe was attacked with an hæmorrhagia uterina

uterina to fo exceffive a degree, that her
life was in imminent danger; and although fhe received every medical affiftance, it was not till after fix weeks from
its commencement, that the flux was totally abated.   After this, tonics were adminiftered, and fhe recovered her bodily
ftrength : but from that period fhe obvioufly became more deranged in her fenfes
than ever fhe had been before.

In the month of April 1775, eleven
months from the commencement of her
diforder, I was confulted by her relations,
who foon afterwards configned her intirely
to my care.   She was in the day-time very
flighty, inconfiftent, vociferous, and loud;
alternately finging, crying, penfive, and
melancholy ; or, as the poet finely de-
picts it,

" In moody madnefs laughing wild,
" Amidft fevereft woe :"

And at night noify, watchful, and turbulent.   The remains of a good conftitution
were very vifible.   As the ftate of her
diforder juftified bleeding, eight ounces of
blood were taken from her arm, on the

eighth

eighth day after her admiffion to my houfe;
the fizy appearance of which induced
me to adminifter to her the volatile and
neutral falts, and a lenient purgative of
the kali tartarifat. and manna, which
from the attendant fymptoms, appeared
moft requifite. From miftaken tendernefs
fhe had long been intemperately indulged. It fhould be remembered, that thofe
who have been accuftomed to command,
cannot obey without the greateft reluctance; and though reafon no longer dif-
criminates between what is right and
wrong, proper and improper; yet the
friends and relatives of maniacs feldom
interpofe, until mifchief occurs from the
omiffion, by the patient being ungovernable through the increafed malignity of the
diforder. Indulgence has always been productive of worfe confequences than would
originate from feafonable reftraint. This
was amply exemplified in the prefent
cafe; for fcarcely any thing to eat or
drink that fhe defired, however irritating
or improper, had been denied; and to
fupprefs her wifhes, however extravagant
and

and unreasonable, would have been deemed by her relations, a most unpardonable relaxation from duty. Thus absurd and injurious are the ideas of their indulgent relations to patients, labouring under such mental pressure. This woman had manifestly been injured by cordials, wines, visitors, and irregular diet. It therefore became absolutely necessary she should abstain from each of these, as the only probable chance of removing the cause, and facilitating the return of her senses. Accordingly, a cool and spare diet was substituted, and a seton passed between the shoulders, in the direction of the spine; a purging draught of kali tartarif. and manna was administered, with a suitable regimen, every third day; and on the intermediate days, the camphorated mixture and nitre in proper proportions, three times in twenty-four hours. After a few weeks, she became manifestly better both in body and mind. Soon succeeding this improvement, she was suddenly seized with rigors, nausea, and thirst, which terminated in an intermittent fever, for which we had
recourse

recourfe to emetics and the cortex, and
every plan of treatment was adopted which
the different indications rendered neceffary,
until the complaint reverted into a continued form. This, by antimonial and antiphlogiftic remedies was foon reduced,
when the bark and nitre in conjunction
were adminiftered, until the patient attained a convalefcent ftate. It was obfervable, that during the attack fhe had
never fhewn any fymptoms of mental derangement, and as her intellectual faculties were at beft but feeble and limited, the
reafon fhe now poffeffed induced her relations to remove her to her own houfe,
where for fome months fhe was afflicted
with a flow nervous fever, but continued
exempt from mania till the time of her
death, which happened about a year and
a half afterwards.

CASE

CASE XXI.

M. P. a lady naturally of a fcorbutic
conftitution, foon after a critical change of
life that occurred to her in her forty-
eighth year, was feized with fpafmodic af-
fe&tions in various parts of her body, great
anxiety, deje&tion, fwelled ankles, faintings,
and difficulty of breathing; from which
complaints, by proper affiftance, fhe was
greatly relieved: but her intelle&tual faculties, that had before been fufceptible of the
moft gentle, delicate, and tender affe&tions,
were foon difcovered to be confiderably
impaired and deranged. Her tafte and
hearing were incorre&t; her eyes pro-
truded and gliftened; fhe fometimes con-
du&ted herfelf with propriety, and fometimes not; till at length fhe became penfive, dull, and thoughtful; and without
any regard to her accuftomed decency,
talked inceffantly, and raved on various
fubje&ts, in fudden tranfitions, as different
images occurred to her diftempered imagination. She had feldom any appetite;
and

and would fometimes, with the greateft
obftinacy, abftain from every kind of fuftenance, with a view, as fhe declared, to
ftarve herfelf by this unnatural perfeverance. After two or three days fevere
abftinence, this refolution forfook her, and
fhe would take any kind of nourifhment
that was left within her reach; but would
neither eat or drink before any perfon
whatever, and always denied that fhe had
taken any food, although it was very obvious that no other perfon had difpenfed
with it. After fhe had thus proved that
fhe had no intention of deftroying herfelf
by this means, fhe feemed obftinately determined on felf-deftruction by other methods, and would certainly have effected
it, in fome way or other, had not the
ftricteft guard been placed over her conduct.

When I firft faw her, I think there
never was a countenance more deeply
impreffed with grief, horror, and melancholy. Her breath was fœtid; fhe had
large, livid, and black fpots, particularly
on her legs and feet; her ankles were
fwelled

fwelled and œdematous; her countenance bloated and fallow. There was a general weaknefs throughout her whole frame. Her tongue was white and rough; fhe had a peculiar degree of rednefs about her noftrils; and her eye-lids were puffed; her fkin was fqualid and dry; and although fhe did not complain of thirft, yet it was very obvious by the eagernefs with which fhe drank. Her fpeech was quick and incoherent; fhe had made but little urine for fome time paft; did not perfpire in the leaft, and was very coftive.

A very tedious hiftorical and uninterefting detail of her cafe was given to me by her hufband; and although it is unneceffary to follow him through every particular circumftance of his narrative, yet I fhall take the liberty to remark, that from his own teftimony the part he had acted with regard to the unfortunate fufferer, had been highly reprehenfible. This juftified fome reports that had been propagated to his difhonour; and if faithfully repeated, reflect but little credit on his conjugal feelings. But as remarks of

G   this

this nature do not come within the com-
pafs of my prefent defign, I fhall revert
to the melancholy objeƈt of my recital,
who was now entirely under my care and
direƈtion, and was removed from a moift
to a dry and pure air. It was evident
that both the folids and fluids were affeƈted by the fcorbutic taint ; therefore the
antifcorbutic juices, with antifeptics, were
adminiftered with good effeƈt ; and the
excretions by perfpiration, urine, and
ftool, were promoted. Her nights were
foothed by the exhibition of fifteen grains
of the faponaceous pill ; which was alfo
attended with the excellent effeƈt of paci-
fying her in the day-time ; her general
diet was that of eafy digeftion, and confifted chiefly of a proper mixture of animal and vegetable fubftances. By this
procefs, in about two months time, the
patient refumed an entirely different countenance, and her intelleƈts were much
relieved : but the remembrance of former troubles feemed to rankle in her
mind ; and notwithftanding fhe converfed
with confiftency, and appeared arduous

to

to conceal her diftrefs, yet the latent
thorn of mental woe was too perceptible.
The medicines and regimen were continued to the end of four months.   When
the putrefactive diathefis feemed to be
perfectly corrected, we had recourfe to
chalybeates, and the cold bath, by which
method the cure of the body and mind
feemed in great meafure effected.

Thus was this patient refcued from the
grave, and reftored to her family; but
this was only a temporary extenfion from
affliction, for a few months after, from
ungentle treatment, and fhameful neglect,
fhe experienced a relapfe, which terminated in fuicide.

―――――――――

CASE XXII.

IN the beginning of the year 1777,
Mrs. E. about forty-two years of age,
was feized with a rigor, reftleffnefs, laffitude, and pain about the loins; to thefe
fymptoms fucceeded exceffive internal

heat,

heat, with great thirft, and an eruption of the eryfipelous kind over all the neck, face, and breaft. Thefe after a few days were fubdued by an antiphlogiftic plan of medicine. But an inftability of mind was foon after obvious in a peculiar caft of her countenance ; fhe talked and imagined ftrange things, was confufed in her ideas, and laboured under much imaginary fear and diftrefs ; which induced her relations to fend her for advice and affiftance to London, where after continuing four months under the care of an eminent phyfician, fhe returned home apparently better, and without any fymptom of maniacal affeciion ; but in the autumn following fhe was attacked with an intermittent fever, which at that time was very frequent in the neighbourhood where fhe refided : this was attended with lofs of appetite, bad digeftion, reftlefs nights, pains in the ftomach and bowels, vapours, and wind.

Her complaints were attributed to a ceffation of the menfes, which had never been very confiderable ; but which had

now

now for fome months entirely ceafed. She complained of pain and tenfion of the tonfils, dimnefs of fight, a flight degree of deafnefs, lofs of ftrength, painful cramp in her legs, lofs of recollection, vertigo, pains in the head and loins, naufea, low-nefs of fpirits, and a general relaxation. All thefe fymptoms had been much ag-gravated by the officious zeal of a perfon of her own fex, who confidered it reli-gioufly neceffary that fhe fhould frequent-ly take hiera picra fteeped in gin—an indifcriminate practice with women in general, to which perfons of nervous and irritable habits often fall victims, through the advice and recommendation of fome Lady Doctor of their acquaintance. A moft violent inflammation of the fauces, eryfipe-las, and piles, fucceeded, with a flight aber-ration of reafon, and diftrefs of mind.

At this period I was confulted, and finding that the patient had a full, hard pulfe, heat, and the above-mentioned fymptoms, I took fix ounces of blood from her arm; and with the affiftance of nitrous

nitrous medicines and gentle aperients, in
a few days relieved her in every refpect,
except the intermittent fever, which foon
after gave way to emetics and a decoction
of nitre and peruvian bark; but fhe foon
after reverted into her former difeafed ftate
of mind, when it became neceffary to
place her more immediately under my
care.   She was inclined to coftivenefs,
was fick at the ftomach, hyfterical, and
yellow in the face.   An antimonial emetic
was given her, which emptied the ftomach
of a great quantity of bile; and as the
beft remedy for her coftivenefs, magnefia
and the lac fulphuris were combined.
The warm pediluvium was ufed every
night and morning; fhe was kept quiet
on a light and nutritive diet, with medicines beft adapted to palliate or relieve
her complaints.   A feton being objected
to, iffues were opened in her legs, and in
a few weeks fhe was entirely free from all
bodily complaints, and poffeffed of her
rational faculties as ufual; but has at times
been troubled with affections of the
                                            nerves,

nerves, from the peculiar nature of her conftitution, and is very fubject to flying pains in her head and ftomach.

CASE XXIII.

MRS. E. H. of a florid complexion, full habit, and remarkable for the fize of her head, at about the age of forty-eight, had for fome time been made a profelyte to a prevailing fyftem of religion, that like an epidemic difeafe had long fpread its baneful influence through many ranks of people, to the excitement of the moft daring outrages, and the wildeft extravagancies. The difciples of this pernicious doctrine, to ufe the words of a very fenfible writer, "are puzzled with their
" own wild fancies; they defert the plain
" and fimple paths of the gofpel, and fel-
" dom infift on thofe things which all may
" underftand, and in which all are greatly
" interefted, that they may feed the fancy
" with an unintelligible jargon, and per-
" plex

" plex the brain : but fuch doctrines will
" never enlighten the underftanding, af-
" fect the heart, or have the fmalleft ten-
" dency to make men either wifer or bet-
" ter. They appear outwardly righteous,
" but within are full of hypocrify and
" iniquity. The terrors of the Lord, and
" the doctrine of a future ftate of rewards
" and punifhments, are proper fubjects on
" feafonable occafions ; but to deal gene-
" rally on fuch fubjects, have a dreadful
" effect on weak minds. Men conftantly
" converfant on gloomy fubjects, naturally
" contract a gloomy and uncharitable
" fpirit ; they banifh gratitude and cheer-
" fulnefs ; they poifon all the fources of
" rational pleafure. Religion, under their
" reprefentation, which fhould be the
" comfort of man, becomes a bondage.
" The God of the Methodifts is not the
" God and Father of our Lord Jefus
" Chrift ; their God is the object of fear,
" not of love. He is reprefented as in-
" throned in heaven, delighting in the
" punifhment of his weak and helplefs
" creatures ; not furrounded with mercy,
                                    " fympa-

" fympathizing with our infirmities; mak-
" ing all gracious allowance for our im-
" perfections, and rejoicing in every re-
" turning prodigal. No profpect can be fo
" difcouraging to man. Religion, defigned
" for the exaltation of our nature, over-
" whelms him with gloomy apprehenfions
" and fear. Religion, which fhould make
" man cheerful, overfpreads him with
" melancholy!"

The defign of this abftract will, I truft,
fufficiently apologize for its infertion,
whilft I proceed to obferve, if it be
true that inftances of infanity are at this
day more numerous in this kingdom than
at any former period, we have abundant
reafon not only to attribute the principal
caufe of it to the prefent univerfal diffufion
of wealth and luxury through almoft every
part of the kingdom; but alfo in fupport
of this opinion to obferve, that fo humi-
liating a degradation of our reafoning faculties owes much of its acceffion to the
abfurd and ill-founded prejudices of that
epidemic enthufiafm, which naturally ex-
cites the attention of weak minds to the
difcuffion of religious points, which they

too

too eagerly contemplate, without the power of clear comprehenfion, to the entire
fubverfion of their intellectual difcern-
ment. Amongft this defcription was the
unfortunate fubject of this cafe; religious
ftudies having fo far gained the afcendency
over her reafon, as to impel her to words
and actions of a maniacal tendency. She
had been taught and imbibed a fixed belief of the manifeftations and interference
of the Deity in her behalf, although her
moral conduct fhould be ever fo reproach-
able or criminal. Tenets fo flattering to
the bafenefs and depravity of the human
heart, as the author of the foregoing quotations juftly obferves "that promife fo
" much, and require fuch fmall facrifices
" of importance, bid fair to be greedily
" embraced, and to become very popular
" among people, who wifh to gain future
" happinefs without any material change
" of their lives."

In this dangerous ftate of fanaticifm fhe
was committed to my care. She had always been ufed to a pretty liberal table;
and as abftemioufnefs had not been among
the

the number of her pretenfions to falvation, fhe had indulged herfelf rather too
freely in the ufe of fpirituous and malt
liquors. A total fuppreffion of the menftrual evacuation had, I was informed,
taken place about two years prior to my
acquaintance with the cafe, when by the
judicious treatment of her apothecary,
fhe had experienced but little interruption of health from the change wrought
upon the conftitution by this law of nature, often productive of the greateft danger; and to which, for the want of proper
advice and affiftance, many an amiable
female has fallen a victim. In the prefent
mode of cure, fhould it be inquired why
I confidered depletion as an indifpenfible appendix, the patient having apparently no bodily complaint to encounter,
I truft that I am juftified in anfwering,
that it is a rule which fhould always be
obferved, when the circulating fluids are
more abundant than is congenial to health,
either from high living, or the fuppreffion
of fome accuftomed evacuation, as was
the cafe with this patient. It had obvioufly

oufly a tendency to increafe the maniacal excitement to a higher pitch than it other-wife would have been. In lefs than two months after fhe had been accuftomed to an abftemious diet, three times bled, and taken laxative dofes of the kali tartar. at fuitable intervals, her blood flowed in a cooler channel, and there was an obvious abatement of the wild antics, religious reveries, and fanatic declamations to which fhe had been fubject; and in a great meafure to be attributed to her fanctified fectaries not having it in their power to procure accefs to her perfon as ufual. No one being permitted to pay the leaft attention to her enthufiaftic exta-fies and raptures, they began gradually to lofe their influence on her mind; and in about eight months appeared to be nearly forgotten. Her reafon being thus com-pletely reftored, fhe returned home to her family, who carefully guarded againft a future relapfe by a firm and fteady refo-lution to prohibit the vifits of thofe zealous devotees, through whofe principles fhe derived the firft impreffion of her terrible affliction. .

CASE

CASE XXIV.

Miss A. P. a young lady who had always been remarkably healthy, one evening after overheating herself by walking,
imprudently drank a large draught of
cold water, and sat down upon a damp
seat in the open air. Very early next
morning she was taken with a pain in her
head and back, attended with rigors, restlessness, anxiety, and intense heat. She
complained of loss of memory, dimness of
sight, weakness, and lassitude; and these
were succeeded by a failure of speech and
delirium. The family physician was immediately consulted; and by bleeding,
blistering, and proper remedies, she was
in some degree recovered; but the attack
was too severe to be entirely subdued, and
left a train of nervous complaints. About
the usual term of her menstruation, she
complained of violent pain in her head,
loins, back, and legs; with pain and palpitation at the navel, spasms at the stomach, and a slow fever. Soon afterwards
she

fhe began to exhibit feveral antic tricks
and geftures, difplayed an uncommon
propenfity to talk, and became bewildered
with fo many ftrange whims and fancies
as to leave no doubt of the brain being in
a difordered ftate. The period above-
mentioned was paffed over without its
ufual falutary effects; nor could all the
advice and management of her friends
procure her any relief or affiftance. She
continued in this ftate near feven months,
and about the end of that time I received
her as a patient into my houfe.

The difeafe itfelf appeared obvioufly to
have arifen in confequence of a contraction of the uterine veffels, from taking
cold. To relieve and relax the parts, the
fteam of warm camphorated water was
ufed, and the warm pediluvium, for nearly
five weeks, before they had the defired
effect. The internal medicine ufed on
this occafion was as follows :

R Calomel. gr. ij.
   Extract Sabinæ gr. iiij.
   Syr. e Mecon. q. f. ut f. Bol.

Which

Which was adminiftered every third evening upon going to bed, drinking a cup of
ftrong horfe-radifh tea, which was alfo repeated alone every fix hours on the intermediate days. We had not continued this
plan longer than the time above-mentioned, when the catamenia returned, her
ideas became progreffively lefs deranged,
and fhe recovered her proper reafon;
which by due care and attention to the
menftrual periods, fhe has ever fince poffeffed without diforder or interruption.

CASE XXV.

THE epidemic catarrh, more generally known by the name of the Influen-
za, which raged with fuch violence in
different parts of the kingdom in the year
1782, prevailed almoft univerfally among
the inhabitants of a town where the patient of whom I am about to fpeak, was
one of the number of the fick. There
was from the firft attack fomething extraordinary

ordinary in her cafe; particularly a ftrange
alteration in her conduct and behaviour,
a tremulous motion of the eyelids, and
little fleep. A flight alienation of mind,
and weaknefs of judgment, were obferved
to accompany the common fymptoms of
the diforder; fhe had fever, and an acute
pain in her head, and at the pit of the
ftomach, with total lofs of appetite, colic
pain, tenfion, and pulfation of the abdomen. The refpiration was quick and difficult; fhe had a flight dry cough, without
expectoration; vain efforts to vomit, attended with diarrhæa, palpitation of the
heart, anxiety, and frequent faintings.
She was bled and bliftered, had fmall dofes
of tartarifed antimony, and was treated
with every degree of medical precifion.
On a remiffion of the febrile fymptom, the
cinchona was given; but this not proving effectual, and great lownefs of fpirits
with cough continuing, fœtid gums and
pectorals were adminiftered, from the effects of which fhe derived fome benefit;
but her fpirits became irregular, and her
mind was not clear and collected; and
for

for some months at intervals slight and transient deviations from reason were observed, till at length the symptoms of insanity were confirmed by deranged and confused ideas, an absence of shame, ridiculous aversions, and unreasonable marks of disgust, hatred, fear, and distress.

She became my patient in the month of August 1783; before which time her menstruations had for six months recurred in slighter quantity than is usual. She laboured under much bodily inquietude, her eyes were protuberant and glistening, their lids much puffed up and slightly inflamed, the pupils unusually distended, and her countenance was pale, bloated, and sickly; she continually muttered to herself, or talked in a vague and incoherent manner; bestowing but little attention upon the objects around. Her cough was not so frequent, but continued very dry and troublesome; she breathed with some degree of difficulty, and several dusky yellowish spots were observed on her arms, legs, and different parts of her body. She was considerably wasted with pain, anxiety, and disorder;

H   and

and before she came to me, she had obtained but little sleep.

Her complaints had frequently been
considered as wholly originating in the
scurvy, a disorder which had been long
hereditarily attached to the family; she
had for some time drank very plentifully of a decoction of the water-dock,
and used every other means appropriate
to that disorder, without success. Her
regimen had never been properly regulated since her illness, and she had been
too much indulged in the use of spirituous
liquors; which had an obvious tendency
to increase her complaint. Her diet now
consisted chiefly of vegetable substances,
with milk; and her general drink was
small white wine whey, or barley water,
with gum arabic and sugar, acidulated
with lemon juice; and the kali acetatum
was given to promote the secretions, combined with the æthiops mineral. Camphor and musk were given every evening
at bed-time in a bolus, and a blister was
applied to the pit of the stomach, which
was kept open a considerable time. This
plan

plan of treatment was continued upwards of four months, with very little variation; and was attended with the happy effect of reftoring the patient to her priftine health and mental confiftency.

———————

CASE XXVI.

IN the year 1776, the parifh officers of Friendfbury applied to me for advice in the cafe of a maniacal patient confined in their workhoufe. This unhappy object had been very defperate, and had committed many acts of outrage and violence; was naturally of a ftrong, mufcular fhape, and rendered much ftronger by his prefent complaint. He had overpowered almoft every one before they could properly fecure him, which was now effected in a very extraordinary manner. He was faftened to the floor by means of a ftaple and an iron ring, which was tied to a pair of fetters about his legs, and he was hand-cuffed. The place of his con-

H 2   finement

finement was a large lower room, occafionally made ufe of for a kitchen, and
which opened into the ftreet; there were
wooden bars to the windows, through the
fpaces of which continual vifitors were
obferving, pointing at, ridiculing, and irritating the poor maniac, who thus became
a fpectacle of public fport and amufement; and by feveral feats of dexterity,
fuch as threading a needle with his toes,
and many other unaccountable tricks and
antics, he had fo far attracted the notice of the public, as feldom to be without
a croud of idle fpectators at the door and
windows of his apartment; and frequently
from the miftaken kindnefs of this inattentive group, he obtained beer, gin, and other
liquors, which ferved to aggravate and inflame his complaint, and keep him in a
conftant ftate of agitation and excitement.

I was requefted to take him immediately home to my houfe; but as the poor
wretch was in a highly infuriate ftate, and
that in great meafure occafioned by the
unfuitablenefs of his fituation, my advice
was to take off his fhackles, and fecure
him

him in a ftrong ftrait-waiftcoat, either of
leather, or of the ftrongeft ticking. Being
informed, however, that this kind of fecurity had been tried, and found ineffectual,
from his gnawing holes in the fhoulders,
and by that means getting his arms loofe,
and the waiftcoat entirely off; to prevent
this in future, I gave directions to have
that part of the waiftcoat which covered
his fhoulders, quilted with brafs wire over
fome fheet lead, and to keep the exterior
parts properly moiftened, from time to
time, with a brufh dipped in a ftrong folution of common aloes; it was alfo my
advice to have a fmall hovel built for his
folitary refidence, in the moft remote part
of the premifes, at a diftance from the
workhoufe, and to prohibit all perfons
from going near enough to converfe with
him, but thofe who fhould be appointed
to the charge of attending him. Befides
this, I directed the furgeon, who had the
fuperintendance of the poor, to keep his
head clofely fhaved, to bleed him *ad deli-*
quium, and repeat the operation as occafion might require; to give him emetics

at

at ftated times, and to keep his body in a
proper ftate of laxity with the kali tartarifat. quickened with the pulvis helle-
bori albi.   Thefe inftructions were effectually put into practice; and proper attention being thus paid to his perfon and
diet, in a few weeks the patient intirely
recovered his reafon ; and begging hard
to be releafed from his confinement, after
I had been again confulted, it was granted,
when he quietly and regularly returned
to his labour and employment; and I
have not heard of his having had any
relapfe.

C A S E   XXVII.

From fome original defect in the conftitution, the fubject of the following recital had from her infancy been difpofed to
cutaneous affections, which appeared in
patches or fpots of an anomalous appearance, and chiefly of a dark colour, on various parts of the body, and were always
attended

attended with a great deal of itching and
heat ; and fhe had fometimes been taken
from fchool, upon the fuppofition that
thefe eruptions had been infectious.
When I was firft confulted, fhe had feveral of thefe blotches upon her arms, legs,
face, and breaft : thofe on the latter parts
greatly refembled a rafpberry, or a mul-
berry, and thofe on the former were of a
whitifh colour, fcaly, dry, and rough.
Mercurials, and other alterative medicines, had been given fome time by the
advice of a regular practitioner, which
operated only as palliatives, and the diforder difappeared and returned fo often,
and the cure became fo hopelefs, that recourfe was had to an itinerant empiric,
who by a fudden repulfion of the humour
for fome weeks, had the credit of having
wrought a moft miraculous cure : but unhappily for the poor patient, much mifchief lurked under this flattering appearance.   On a fudden, her imagination was
difturbed, which was vifible in the countenance, voice, and gefture; and a ftrange
alteration was perceived in her manner
and

and behaviour. The firſt ſigns of her
alienation of mind were diſcovered about
the uſual return of the catamenia, when
ſhe became furious, turbulent, and audacious; but was afterwards more dejected,
penſive, and timorous; and often waked
out of her ſleep in moſt outrageous fits of
violence and paſſion. She complained of
cephalalgic pains, riſings in the throat, and
ſpaſms at the pit of the ſtomach, which
continued violent and without intermiſſion.
Her countenance was moroſe, gloomy, and
ſorrowful; her eyes were wild and pro-
truded; their pupils much dilated, and
her complexion ſallow and cachectic.
She was bled, had a bliſter between her
ſhoulders, and another at the ſcrobiculus
cordis. The pulſe was hard and ſmall;
her reſpiration deep and ſlow. She apparently grew worſe, refuſed all kind of
food, and ſhewed an obſtinate propenſity
to ſuicide; from the perpetration of which
horrid action ſhe was with difficulty reſtrained.

At this period I was firſt conſulted,
when ten weeks had elapſed ſince the laſt

                                        return

return of the catamenia. Every word
and action betrayed the moft violent agitation of mind, which it was not in her
own power to amend or correct; fhe was
always intent upon one fubject; delir-
ous without fever, and ftedfaftly bent upon her own deftruction; which rendered
it highly incumbent upon thofe about
her to exert their utmoft care and dili-
gence to prevent her terrible defign.
The kali tartarifat. was given her in the
quantity of three drachms every fecond
or third day; a thin diet and diluting
drinks, with the ufe of the warm bath,
were ordered every night and morning;
a feton was made between her fhoulders,
and the pediluvium not omitted; and to
recover the menftrual evacuations, the
following pills were adminiftered twice a
day:

R Extract Sabinæ   ʒifs.
  Pulv. e Myrrha C. ʒfs.
  Kali pp.   gr. xv.
  Syr. S. q. f. ut f. Pil. mediocr.

Befides which, forty drops of the tinct.
ferri muriata were given every morning in
a cup-

a cupful of infufum raphan. ruftic. rad. and repeated in the afternoon at five o'clock ; and as proper evacuants had preceded, occafionally a fmall quantity of the tinct. opii camphorat. was given at bed-time, which rendered her nights much eafier.

In a few weeks the menfes returned, fhe recovered her appetite; and her countenance, from being gloomy, pallid, and contracted, became more natural, lively, and open ; the eruption to which fhe had fo long been fubject, re-appeared on her forehead, cheeks, and breafts ; but was obferved to be of a more florid hue than ufual ; and the patient having recovered her reafon, it was judged unneceffary to make any farther attempts to conquer a diforder that feemed interwoven in the conftitution, and which all endeavours to expel had proved of fo dangerous a tendency.

CASE

CASE XXVIII.

IMMERSED in the deepeſt abyſs of melancholy, which had produced an univerſal muſcular decay, Mr. B. B. was put under my care in the month of July 1777. He was naturally of a choleric habit, and of a violently paſſionate diſpoſition. His eyes were full, bright, and protuberant; and he was ſubject to flatulencies in the abdomen. His anxiety was inexpreſſible; his appetite was ſometimes totally loſt or depraved, and at others preternaturally increaſed: his aſpect was dark and gloomy; he had much conſtipation of the bowels; his breath was hot and offenſive; he was ſurly, moroſe, and dogmatical in his converſation, carriage, and behaviour. His eye-lids were puffed up and ſwelled; he was turbulent, reſtleſs, and unruly; and he had upon him an eruption not unlike the *herpes miliaris,* which appeared in circles over all the neck, back, face, and arms; his pulſe was quick, ſtrong, and hard, with preternatural

ral heat; and his urine was very high coloured.

As very little attention had been paid to his diet, it was become expedient to regulate it upon a plan that was more cooling, light, and nourifhing; and to indulge him lefs liberally in the liquors to which he had been accuftomed. The kali tartarifatum was occafionally adminiftered as a gentle laxative, and a feton was made between his fhoulders. He was three times bled, and camphor with nitre given him every evening at bed-time, and repeated during the night, when reftlefs and uneafy; by which means he daily became better, and progreffively recovered his health and fpirits.

After four months continuance with me, having for fome time enjoyed a lucid interval, he was judged by his relations to be well enough to return home: the refult of which imprudent determination was a relapfe; and he was committed to my care again in lefs than fix weeks, when I again adopted the fame mode of treatment as before, and in a few months was equally fuccefsful.

fuccefsful.   At the inftance of his friends,
another trial was propofed and made,
the confequence of which was (as might
reafonably be expe&ted) a fecond relapfe;
with this difference, however, that I now
totally difclaimed all further concern with
a cafe, where the relations themfelves had
fo little reafon and confideration; and
the unfortunate man was foon after fent to
a mad-houfe at Iflington, where he died
in about a month after his admiffion.

This cafe furnifhes another to the numerous proofs which I could adduce,
demonftrable of the inutility and impro-
priety of removing the convalefcent maniac too foon to his former refidence—a
method of all others the leaft adapted to
the re-eftablifhment of impaired or relaxed intelle&ts.   Domeftic concerns and
fudden preffure of bufinefs obtruding
themfelves on a mind not fufficiently
ftrong and colle&ted to bear fuch im-
preffions, and digeft the recent influx of
ideas naturally occafioned by fuch a
material change of fituation, hurry and
overwhelm the animal fpirits; and a relapfe

lapfe of the moft dangerous kind is always
to be dreaded.

———————

CASE XXIX.

T. B. in the twenty-feventh year of her
age, had the misfortune fuddenly to lofe
a very near relation, which threw her into the moft violent fpecies of delirium,
attended with ravings and a continued
fever; for which a blifter was applied to
the head, a ftimulating cataplafm to her
feet, and antiphlogiftic medicines were
adminiftered. Thefe methods fubdued
the fever, but fhe remained in a forrow-
ful and melancholy fituation, often breaking out into peevifh and angry exclama-
tions; and indeed the whole mode of her
behaviour was obferved to be the very
reverfe of her natural manners and amiable difpofition. Sometimes fhe evinced
a remarkable energy of imagination; at
others fhe would throw herfelf into the
moft violent fits of paffion and ground-

lefs

lefs refentment againft perfons who were
fcarcely known to and had never injured
her.   Thus noify, turbulent, and contentious, fhe was difpofed to every kind of
mifchief that violence and defpair could
poffibly produce.   On this account, for
the fecurity of herfelf and friends, it was
thought neceffary to fecure her in the
ufual manner ; which on account of the
acceffion of ftrength attached to her complaint, was accomplifhed with much difficulty and trouble.   In this ftate fhe almoft continually raved, menaced, fwore,
fcreamed, talked obfcenely, or anfwered
with the moft vehement anger to all about
her, and had little or no fleep by night or
day ; fo that her friends were entirely
wearied out with the inceffant din and
noife which fhe created, and committed
her wholly to my charge.

I difcovered that fhe had a tumour in
the back part of her neck, with an appearance of fuppuration ; her appetite
was depraved ; the abdomen was tenfe
and hard, probably from the long confti-
pation fhe had endured, which had been
                                    for

for the fpace of ten or twelve days; fo
that it might be reafonably expected the
putrid contents of the abdomen had generated a quantity of air: fhe had frequently
fpafmodic contractions of the joints, with
violent pains and convulfions of the whole
frame: her deglutition was very difficult;
fhe difcharged the urine involuntarily;
had frequent eructations; her eyes were fuffufed with blood; the face was contracted;
and a great heat appeared over her whole
body: fhe had a hoarfenefs, with a peculiar hollow and difmal voice. The cuti-
cle was tinged with a yellow dye; and fhe
had often a palpitation of the heart, attended with extreme pain and anxiety.
And here I may be allowed to obferve
with Dr. Battie, that though the brain is
undoubtedly the feat of delufive fenfation,
neverthelefs it is not the only one; for-
afmuch as fanguinary or ferous obftructions in other parts are capable of exciting
falfe ideas, in proportion to the medullary
matter collected, fo as to be compreffed
by fuch obftructions. Thus the ftomach,
inteftines, and uterus, are frequently the
real

real feats of madnefs, occafioned by the
contents of thefe vifcera being obftructed
in fuch a manner as to comprefs the many
nervous filaments which here communicate with one another by the mefenteric
ganglia.

To remove her obftinate coftivenefs,
an emollient clyfter was ufed; but not
having the defired effect, another of a
more ftimulating nature, was adminiftered,
which after a confiderable time anfwered
the purpofe.   I then gave her an emetic,
confifting of

> Vin. Ipec. ℥j.
> Antimon. Tart. gr. j.

which brought away a furprizing quantity of crude bile.   A feton was made
between her fhoulders in the direction of
the fpine, below the bafis of the tumour;
fhe was occafionally purged with the kali
tartarifatum, &c.   The tinctura fuliginis
was given her three times a day, in the
quantity of thirty or forty drops in a cupful of the camphorated mixture.   A ftrict
attention was paid to cleanlinefs; her re-

gimen was duly regulated; and after a
perfeverance of nearly four months, her
health and reafon being pretty well eftablifhed, fhe returned to her relations;
and I believe has never fince had any return of infanity, although the feton has
been healed long fince, and every other
remedy difcontinued.

CASE XXX.

A Lady of the moft diftinguifhed lite-
rary abilities, and who at all times has
proved herfelf obligingly ready to bear
grateful teftimony to the truth of thefe
premifes, applied to me on the fifth of
May 1779, concerning her brother, a
dignified clergyman in this county, who
for twelve months paft had laboured under a privation of fpeech and fenfes, icte-
rical affections, and nervous debility.
From the beginning of his complaint he
had been attended by two eminent practitioners. He was about eight-and-forty
years

years of age, and had in the earlier part of
life been attacked with the gout in his
feet, which continued for a fortnight, and
fometimes longer.   Some time before his
prefent diforder he had fymptoms of indigeftion, complained of obtufe pain in
the left hypochondrium, and fometimes of
tenfion and weight in the region of the
heart, extending to the loins and bladder,
and frequently recurring with an extenfion to the head, neck, ftomach, and
bowels, accompanied with an almoft continual naufea and acid eructations ; for
which he had taken an emetic, and finding
fome relief, ftomachic medicines and warm
purgatives had fucceeded.

The fymptoms he laboured under were
imputed to the latent gout; and for want
of a regular fit, in fupport of this opinion,
proper methods had been purfued to
bring on a paroxyfm of that diforder;
but not being effected, and no fubftantial
benefit derived from this treatment, faponaceous and aloetic medicines were
given him; from which for fome time
it was thought that he received affift-
I 2   ance;

ance : but his former fymptoms recurring, with the addition of coftivenefs, dejection, and melancholy, I was defired to vifit him, and to give my opinion of his cafe to his relations. He was then at a village in the vicinity of the metropolis, attended by two affiftants who never left him. From the gentleman of the houfe where he boarded, I received the following relation, " That he never offered to " drefs or undrefs himfelf; that he never " ate, without being fed like a child; that " he fat whole days together with his eyes " rivetted to the ground; fometimes appeared dejected, fretful, and timorous; " and at others was fo furious in his manner " and gefture as to render coercion abfo- " lutely neceffary; that his eyes were in " general heavy and fixed; their coats " tinged with yellow, and often red and " inflamed; he was fubject to troublefome " flatulencies, inexpreffible anxiety in the " day time, and was reftlefs and watchful " at nights, but never uttered a word; " was generally coftive; his urine thin " and in fmall quantities. He often " fetched

" fetched deep fighs, and drew his breath
" with difficulty; had fometimes a flufh-
" ing in his cheeks, at others a livid co-
" lour, with a dull, dark, and ftupid
" afpect; fudden ftools and fhaking of
" the whole body; and that his excre-
" ments were in general indurated, and of
" a red colour, or covered with yellow
" bile; that when fpoken to, he appeared
" in a ftate of torpidity; his eye-lids were
" puffed; in fitting he inclined to the right
" fide, placing his hand on the left, as if
" he felt pain in the left hypochondrium,
" which on examination was found to be
" tenfe and hard; a yellownefs was dif-
" fufed over his whole body, which would
" often difappear for four or five days, or
" a week at a time, and then re-appear;"
a circumftance (it may be obferved) not
very uncommon in many hypochondriacal
and maniacal cafes.   To this account was
added, " That his urine was made at long
" intervals; appeared to be voided with
" difficulty, and was in general of a whey
" colour, thin, limpid, and pale; nor had
" ever any fediment been obferved in it
                                    " but

" but once, which was foon after the ope-
" ration of a ftrong emetic, when it was
" faid to be much charged with bile."

The pulfe was hard, quick, and full.
He appeared of a truly atrabilious habit,
and as fenfelefs as a ftatue. Under the
influence of this fullen taciturnity, his
figure and fituation brought to my remembrance the lines fo beautifully defcriptive of a melancholy maniac.

" ————— When gloomy the black bile prevails,
" And lumpifh phlegm the thicken'd mafs congeals,
" All lifelefs then is the poor patient found,
" And fits for ever mufing on the ground.
" His active powers their ufes all forego,
" Nor fenfes, tongue, nor limbs their ufes know.
" In melancholy loft, the vital flame
" Informs, and juft informs, the liftlefs frame."

Without attempting the inveftigation
of a cafe, which in its nature was too ab-
ftracted and complicated for the practitioner to deduce any conclufions that
could be in the leaft degree certain or
fatisfactory, I ventured only to adopt
fuch an hypothefis, as from the nature of
the circumftances, might probably in fome
degree

degree be fuccefsful; and notwithftanding the pitiable and almoft hopelefs fituation which he was reduced to, fuch was
the opinion which was entertained of my
judgment, that I was defired to render
him every medical affiftance in my power,
and attend daily on his perfon; a tafk
which, I moft candidly declare, was un-
dertaken with the utmoft diffidence and
with the moft forlorn hope of fuccefs. To
awaken, as it were, and to roufe him from
this ftate of apathy, and accelerate the
natural action of the fyftem, feemed to
be the moft probable indications of cure:
repeated phlebotomy, blifters, a feton, the
warm pediluvium, volatile embrocations
to the left fide, fomentations to the feet and
leg, emetics at ftated periods, the warm
bath, cupping with and without fcarification, electricity, laxative dofes of ol. ricini,
camphorated mixture with volatiles at
bed-time, James's powders, and fuch other
medicines as feemed likely to promote
the fecretions, were alternately and inef-
fectually ufed for the fpace of eighteen
months, without producing any material
alteration

alteration or effect. The emetics generally confifted of ant. tartarifat. gr. iij. and
feldom failed to evacuate a quantity of
dark-coloured bile from the ftomach. The
fteams of warm water, in which rofemary,
myrrh, vinegar, and camphor were mixed,
were conftantly diffufed two or three times
a day, over the head and face for fifteen
and twenty minutes at a time, and warm
fpirituous applications were ufed as fomentations to the extremities, without the
leaft favourable prognoftic or refult.

Wearied with fo long and fruitlefs an
attendance, and the cure ftill continuing
an object of doubtful hope and fearful uncertainty, I requefted to be difmiffed from
my appointment, and recommended that
a trial might be made of fuch practitioners whofe fkill and judgment were
fanctioned by longer practice than my
own, which though perhaps eafily to
be found, I flattered myfelf not one
could be found whofe affiduity and defire
to ferve the patient could be more
fteady and fincere. Of this his friends
feemed gratefully convinced, and therefore

fore requefted I would continue my
advice and affiftance fome time longer.
In this fecond trial I contented myfelf
with giving him the emetics as before, at
the diftance of every third or fourth week;
and laying afide every other medicine,
made trial of the following mixture:

R Mift. Camphorat.
    Aq. Menth. Piperit. aa. ℥iv.
    Sp. Æth. Vitr. ʒij. M. f. Mift.

which was adminiftered to him in the quantity of a cupful frequently, and was continued four months before its efficacy was the
leaft apparent, when his urine began to
appear turbid, with a fediment; his afpect
gradually unbent and refumed its natural
appearance; he could walk without an
attendant, and without attracting notice
by any fingularity of his gait or manner;
he now perfpired, efpecially towards the
morning; was calm and eafy, and his
fleep refrefhing. After a little time he
began to feed himfelf, and converfe in his
ufual manner, and to take proper exercife. A ftomachic bitter was added to
                        his

his medicine. His ſtools were now natural and regular. He entirely recovered
his fleſh; and about the beginning of
February 1782, he went to Bath, where
he continued about ten weeks, and returned in a very good ſtate of health;
and by a letter replete with the moſt
lively gratitude, with which I was ho-
noured, it gave me the greateſt ſatis-
faƈtion to know that he continued uninterruptedly well, both in body and
mind; and has ever ſince been capable of fulfilling the duties of his function with every degree of propriety,
religiouſly enforced both by precept and
example.

CASE XXXI.

ABOUT ſeven years ago, Miſs E. T.
of Chicheſter, five-and-twenty years of
age, of a tender and delicate conſtitution,
and extreme ſenſibility, without any apparent cauſe whatever, was ſuddenly ſeized
with

with a ftrangulation of the fauces, from
which time fhe became low-fpirited, fuper-
ftitioufly fearful of future occurrences, coftive, and fubject to flatulencies, anxiety,
and violent perturbations of mind. Her
appetite was depraved; fhe had eructations, diftenfion of the ftomach, pain, and
cardialgia. Her ideas were difordered and
incoherent; and at times fhe was fubject
to a kind of epileptic fyncope, in which
for fome minutes fenfation feemed totally
fufpended. The urine was fometimes
fuppreffed for five or fix days together,
and always voided with pain; and was
fometimes obferved to depofit a copious
fediment, mixed with fabulous concretions. She had a dry, frequent cough,
without expectoration, that was much
increafed by motion or fwallowing, and
more particularly fo in the period of
irritation. Her eyes were bright, wild,
full, and projecting; her face was bloated and florid; and every action wildly
lafcivious, abfurd, or extravagant. She
had feldom any febrile heat, but conftantly complained of intenfe pain, alternately

nately in the forehead and back part of the head; and fometimes in the fpine of the back and epigaftric region. The menfes were fuppreffed, and hyfterical faintings frequently fuperfeded.

The beft medical advice was fought; but after many repeated trials, the cafe ftill eluded the efforts of every practitioner that had been confulted. When fent to me, fhe was much emaciated in body, and in a ftate of mind little fhort of raving madnefs; but at intervals fenfible of her diforder. As her madnefs had been of fuch confiderable duration, I entertained not the leaft hope of adminiftering any relief, but from the firft deemed the cafe incurable. Her refpiration was quick and fhort; the cough as before defcribed; her pulfe weak, quick, and hard; fhe had frequent rigors, with reftleffnefs, pain in the loins, contraction, diftortion of the features, and fpafms of the mufcles along the fpine, bending the body backwards. The voice was feeble, and fcarcely articulate; and in fhort, her whole fyftem was fuch as to threaten the moft

fatal

fatal confequence: yet by means of tepid fomentations, expectorants, &c. the cough abated, and her refpiration was relieved. She revived from this alarming ftate, and became fo much better in every refpect, that for fome weeks together hopes were entertained of her entire recovery: but on a fudden, after having paffed a reftlefs night, the cough returned, fhe complained of a ftraitnefs acrofs her breaft, and a great difficulty of breathing enfued, with an œdematous fwelling of the face, arms, hands, and feet: fhe paffed little or no urine, and had conftantly nocturnal febrile fymptoms; but by lofing a fmall quantity of blood, and the free ufe of the powder and oxymel of fquills, all thefe complaints difappeared, but at the inftant when fhe appeared recovering, fhe died fuddenly from fuffocation.

It being a defire that fhe herfelf had frequently expreffed, during her lucid intervals, that her head fhould be opened to difcover the caufe of her complaints, and meeting with the entire concurrence of her friends, it was accordingly performed, when the appearances

pearances were as follow: the right temporal artery was very much enlarged; and on removing the fcull, the brain was extremely turgid, and could not be again returned within the cranium, which was uncommonly thick, efpecially on the *right fide:* the feptum nafi appeared to have experienced fome elongation: the dura mater adhered to the fcull in feveral places; but more particularly fo to the right parietal and occipital bones; and the veffels appeared varicofe: the fubftance of the brain itfelf appeared partially indurated, and the finuffes were every where diftended with blood: the right fide of the pia mater was of a dark livid colour, and fomewhat thickened: the brain, in its general texture, was more flaccid than is ufual: the lateral ventricles contained a quantity of yellowifh fluid: the plexus choroides was in a natural ftate: the pineal gland was larger than common, remarkably foft of texture, and furrounded with a watery fluid: the carotid arteries and jugular veins were preternaturally enlarged: our examination was extended to the thorax and abdomen; in the former

mer

mer of which the appearance differed but little from a natural ſtate, excepting only a veſicular adheſion to the pericardium, which contained a quantity of ſerous fluid: in the latter, the ſtomach appeared in a natural ſtate, excepting the pylorus, which ſeemed to be affeſted with a ſchirrous hardneſs, and was cloſely contraſted: the liver had hydatids on its ſurface, and the ſpleen ſeemed to be unuſually large, but of a natural complexion: the omentum was ſomewhat diſcoloured, in many places adhered to the peritonæum; and the veſſels in general appeared diſtended, and in many parts to have become varicoſe.

Perhaps no true judgment can be formed in theſe caſes from diſſeſtions, as the morbid appearance of the brain has hitherto afforded but little elucidation to diſcover the cauſe of maniacal affeſtions; yet I am of opinion, that it might be of ſome advantage if thoſe gentlemen who have frequent opportunities of diſſeſting the bodies of maniacal patients, were to deſcribe with accuracy the different morbid

bid appearances which prefent themfelves. Perhaps fome information might be derived from weighing the cerebrum and cerebellum of fuch patients, as they have diffected *, and from thence deducing

* Michell, in his Anatomico Phyfiological Refearches into the Caufe of the various Kinds of Infanity which have their Seat in the Body, *(Memoire de l'Academie Royale des Sciences et Belles Lettres, a Berlin,* 1766) fays, that he has difcovered by the moft careful and accurate experiments, that the fpecific gravity of the brain of a melancholy or maniacal patient, is very different from that of the brain of a fane perfon. A cube of fix lines of the brain of a healthy man weighed four, or at the moft fix grains; allowing fome difference from the different ftates of diftenfion in the blood veffels. But in maniacs and melancholic patients, the brain is harder, drier, and more elaftic in its texture, and weighs feven drachms *(Mem. De l'Academie de Berlin, tom. xx. p. 75.)* In addition to this generally difeafed ftate of the brain, particular local alterations may alfo occur; as for inftance, earthy concretions may form in its fubftance from ferous congeftion; from preffure by a larger determination of blood to the brain; from pus, or nervous irritation: but notwithftanding what has been faid, the brain of maniacal fubjects has feldom appeared materially altered, and has often been found not to be in the leaft harder, drier, or more elaftic than is
ufual

deducing such comparative inferences as
should appear interesting or singular: although

usual *(Adversac Med. Pract. Leipsic*, 1769, *tom. viii. P. 3.
p.* 584, *et sequent.)* Having observed that the skull of this
patient was *uncommonly thick* on one side more than the
other, I shall here take the liberty of adding an extract
from the ingenious Dr. Crichton's " Inquiry into the
" Nature and Origin of Mental Derangement," which
immediately applies to this observation. "It is very
" remarkable," he says, "that the skulls of the greater
" number of such patients are commonly very *thick*,
" nay sometimes have been found of an extraordinary
" degree of *thickness*. Among two hundred and sixteen
" patients of this description, whose bodies were in-
" spected after death, there were found one hundred
" and sixty-seven, whose skulls were unusually *thick*,
" and only thirty-eight thin ones; among which last
" number there was one which was much *thicker* on
" the *right* side than the left: but in particular it was
" observed, that among one hundred raving madmen,
" seventy-eight had very *thick* skulls, and twenty very
" *thin* ones; among which skulls there was one quite
" soft. Among twenty-six epileptic raving madmen,
" there were nineteen found with very *thick* skulls, and
" four very thin. Among sixteen epileptic idiots there
" were fourteen, and among twenty epileptic patients
" sixteen, who had very *thick* skulls; among whom
" there was one discovered, one side of whose skull
" was *thick*, and the other thin. Among twenty-four
" melancholic patients, there were eighteen with very

K thin

though it is much to be feared the result of such researches, however ingenious, would fall very short of the desired effect; and the appearance, however diversified, leave the specific nature and the proximate cause of insanity still to dubious hypothesis; and the aberration of our reason remain for ever beyond the reach of human comprehension.

———

CASE XXXII.

COMMUNICATED to me by letter, from Mr. B. Spinluff, Surgeon, of South Heddingham, in Essex.

" Sir,

" I AM requested to write you the case of a lady in this neighbourhood, whose melancholy turn of mind has ren-

———

" thin skulls. And lastly, among thirty idiots, twenty-" two with very *thick,* and six with very thin skulls.
" All the rest had skulls of a natural *thickness.*"

dered

dered her unfit for fociety, and given the
greateft anxiety to her friends and relations.   She is about fixty years of age, or
rather more ; fhe has been affected with a
depreffion of fpirits forty years, which
has fince fettled into a fixed melancholy.
She was at that time conveyed to fome
public hofpital, (I think St. Luke's)
where fhe caught the fmall-pox.   The
puftules were pretty numerous, but diftinct ; and her former complaint very
happily terminated with the latter, and
fhe remained in a tolerable ftate of health
till within the laft two years ; when, as I
am informed, the medical gentlemen declared the fever and complaint in her
bowels, with which fhe was then feized,
was of a bilious nature, and fhe was treated accordingly.   It is to be remaked, that
during her indifpofition, fhe had a flight
falivation, and was then perfectly free from
every diftreffing idea.   No fooner did the
fpitting ceafe, than fhe became low-fpirited, and embarraffed with a continual
train of the moft anxious thoughts.   I
am not able to fay how far the falivation

was occafioned by the mercury exhibited during the bilious complaint, but am inclined to fuppofe it was the effect of it.

I was defired to vifit this unfortunate lady, about a year ago, and found her mind filled with horror, fear, and folicitude; her pulfe quick and full. She was thirfty, and indulged in an unlimited ufe of meat, good ale, and wine. Her urine was fometimes pale and fometimes high coloured, and never depofited any kind of fediment: her appetite was good, and her memory perfect: fhe had feveral hours fleep in the night; yet was apparently more miferable after it. I have taken blood from the arm repeatedly, and given her purgatives and antimonial pills at proper intervals; at the fame time infifting on a cooling diet and diluting liquors, with which fhe has complied, although reluctantly. Since my firft attending her, I have given calomel in fmall dofes, with a view of procuring a flight return of the fpitting; but was never able to obtain what I thought fo defirable a purpofe. The fauces became a little fore, and the breath offenfive,

offenfive, in confequence of the mercury, but not the leaft fpitting: I therefore laid it afide, and had recourfe to the former treatment. She remains rather more compofed, but ftill in an unhappy ftate, and her friends would be glad to do any thing in their power to contribute to her recovery. They beg that you will inform them by letter directed to me, whether you think at her time of life there is any probability of a cure; or if you chufe to order any medicine, they will be ready to make a proper acknowledge-ment.

I am, Sir,

Your humble fervant,

B. SPINLUFF."

S. Heddingham, Effex,
  Nov. 19, 1782.

MY ANSWER.

" Sir,

" THE cafe you mention is a very fingular one indeed; but forty years hav-ing elapfed fince her melancholy com-plaint

plaint firſt took place, is a long ſpace of time. Your conjecture in regard to the mercury is very probable, and founded in judgment; but as the calomel which you have adminiſtered, has not proved efficient in producing a ſalivation, and its internal uſe may perhaps be unfriendly to the primæ viæ, ſuppoſe you were to rub a few grains of it within-ſide the cheek, every night and morning, according to Clare's method of ſalivation, which is eaſily to be raiſed by this means, for proof of which I refer you to his book. It is very probable that a freſh diſcharge from the ſalival glands may be attended with relief; and if you approve of it, would adviſe a trial. Should it not ſucceed, a ſeton I preſume ſhould be the next thing tried. Her -very liberal mode of living muſt throw inſuperable ohſtacles in the way of cure ; a ſlender and cooling regimen ſhould be ſubſtituted, and her body opened with the kali tartar. What was the general complexion and texture of the blood ? I think there is ſome probability of rendering the patient ſervice; and

our

our joint endeavours fhall be directed to
that end : therefore as no good has arifen
from the ufe of venefection, purgatives,
or vomits, let us lay them afide, endeavour
to excite a fpitting with the calomel, and
keep the body in a proper ftate of laxity
with the kali tartarifat. or the ol. ricini,
as befts fuits that purpofe, in fuch dofes
as may be well adapted for that end.   Let
the patient ufe the warm pediluvium,
and immediately afterwards take a cupful
of camphorated mixture, which may be
repeated as often as you think neceffary.
When the anxiety is moft intenfe, reclining the head over the fteams of hot water,
not only affords a temporary relief, but
frequently has a very permanent good
effect.   Frictions with a coarfe towel, or
a flefh brufh, are in thefe cafes very often
ferviceable.   Thefe documents, however,
I fubmit to your confideration; and
fhould they meet with your concurrence,
may be immediately reduced to practice.
If thought neceffary, I can make it convenient to vifit the patient, as fpeaking
often conveys more than writing; but
                                    this

this I leave to the decifion of yourfelf and
the friends of the afflicted lady, and in the
mean time,

I am, &c."

THE REPLY.

"Dear Sir,

"THE uncertainty of our profef-
fion is ever an apology in the line of correfpondence; and you need not be re-
minded that in this refpect we are in
general the leaft to be depended on,
yourfelf only an exception to this remark.
I have to beg pardon for not fooner anfwering your obliging and polite letter,
and have to inform you, that our patient
has conformed beyond expectation to
your advice, and I think has received confiderable benefit. A gentle fpitting fucceeded the abforption of the mercury in
a very agreeable manner, according to
Clare's direction, and which continues as
I could wifh. She feems much compofed
by the immerfion of her feet in warm
water.

water. The camphorated mixture has been given every night, and agrees very well with her. I am this morning writing to the gentleman who has the eſtate, recommending in the ſtrongeſt terms that you might pay her a viſit, as he is a ſenſible good man, and would do any thing for her good; and when favoured with his anſwer, ſhall do myſelf the pleaſure of writing to you again; and find a ſingular ſatisfaction in ſubſcribing myſelf,

Your humble ſervant,

B. SPINLUFF."

S. *Heddingham,*
Jan. 9th, 1783.

CASE XXXIII.

IN March 1779, my advice and aſſiſtance was requeſted by letter in the caſe of J. O. a perſon of great reſpectability, who had ſeveral times been in a very unhappy ſtate of mind; his ſpirits were unuſually exhilarated in ſummer, and as much

much depreffed in winter, owing to a free
way of life to which he had been too much
addicted from his early youth. He was
now upwards of three-and-forty years of
age; and his diforder, which it was hoped
would have gradually decreafed, appeared
in the fummer before, in confequence of
the hurrying life in which he was engaged prior to and at the time of encamp-
ment, with redoubled violence. He was
very indifferent the preceding fpring, and
was attended a few times by a phyfician
in London, who thought (as others of the
faculty had) his cafe to be nervous. Some
had conjectured that the ufe of mercurials
in his younger days had been of differvice
to him; and a variety of caufes had been
affigned for his diforder, which not being
hereditary, (no one of his family having
ever had any thing of the kind) his relations imputed it entirely to his mode of
living, and ftill hoped that it might be
relieved, if not entirely removed.

Notwithftanding this mental infirmity,
he was much beloved by his acquaintance; and when at the worft generally
appeared

appeared to ſtrangers perfectly well. His
appetite was ſmall, and he was either
rigidly coſtive, or lax to an extreme;
drowſy, dejected, forgetful, and ſubject to
acid eructations: he often complained
that he ſaw objects indiſtinctly; was at
times bold and reſolute, or ridiculouſly
timid, fearful, and ſuſpicious; and complained of a head-ach like that which
ariſes from a crowded theatre, and of being hot and thirſty; yet had no actual
fever.   He had frequent pains in the left,
and ſometimes in the right hypochondrium; but without any perceptible tenſion in either.   His digeſtion was very
bad; he ſuffered a general debility of the
whole frame; had diſtreſſing ideas; was
conſcious that the functions of his. mind
were impaired, and was fearful that it
would end in confirmed mania.   His
pulſe was ſlow, weak, and often irregular;
he would frequently fetch deep ſighs, and
fancy his life in imminent danger; he
paſſed reſtleſs and uneaſy nights; his
urine was in general pale, and almoſt colourleſs, forming no cloud, and depoſiting

no

no fediment. The difordered ftate of his mind, as well as body, feemed to originate in the fame caufe ; therefore late hours, drinking in a morning, gay and diffipated company, was abfolutely neceffary to be avoided; a moderate diet and temperate regulation of every kind feemed to pro-mife him the greateft relief. To relieve and affift the alimentary canal, a gentle emetic was prefcribed ; his coftivenefs was relieved by alternate dofes of kali tartar. and ol. ricini, and a fuitable diet; his nights were rendered more eafy by the pil. ftyrace and camphor in a fmall quan-tity, which though not often prefcribed in mania, yet ought not to be totally difcard-ed, as a trial of opium in a fmall degree cannot be very injurious ; and as in this cafe, by diminifhing the irritability, may fometimes prove of fervice. He made ufe of the cold bath, and ftrengthening medi-cines, as moft conducive to the cure of relaxation, with fuccefs; and by an ex-tenfion of temperance in the non-naturals, recovered his former mental vigour and bodily health, in a fpace of time not ex-ceeding

ceeding four months ; and by continuing
fo to do with a manly firmnefs and refolution, he acquired fuch an habitual line
of felf-regulation, as fecured to him that
ftate of body and mind, which it is the wifh
of every man to enjoy and preferve.

CASE XXXIV.

A Lady about thirty years of age, of a
gloomy and referved difpofition, was put
under my care in the year 1784. About
feven years before, fhe had made an attempt to deftroy herfelf, after which fhe
continued well for three years, when fome
little difturbance happening in the family, which no way concerned her, fhe
chofe to take an active part; but the
vexation which occurred from being difappointed in her views, threw her ill
again, and fhe made another attempt
on her life ; upon which her father put
her to board in a family where fhe was
an utter ftranger, and unconnected with
any

any one. She continued well in this fituation two years, but about three months
before fhe came to me, was attacked with
a nervous fever, was deranged in her ideas,
had a wild appearance in her looks, and
was often agitated in the night, fo as fuddenly to ftart up and fly out of the bed.
By proper remedies, however, fhe got
the better of this, but foon relapfed into
the fame deranged fituation, and a third
time attempted to commit fuicide.

In her beft ftate of mind, fhe was a
perfon little fufceptible of gentle, tender, or delicate affections, and of very
narrow and circumfcribed ideas; at this
crifis fhe had the moft repulfive afpect I ever beheld, her appearance ex-
hibiting an exact emblem of her mind.
A fullen taciturnity poffeffed her, and fhe
fcarcely knew or attended to any external
object; her fkin was pale and fallow,
fqualid and dry; the pulfe hard and full;
and her feet and ankles were much fwelled
in the evening.

To excite a ftimulus, electricity was
ufed; and upon taking blood from the
                                      arm,

arm, it exhibited a viscid appearance.
The warm pediluvium was used regularly
every night, and the camphorated mixture given at bed-time, and occasionally
repeated.   Her bowels were kept moderately lax, with an aperient electuary;
and the menstrual discharge, which had
ceased for some time past, was promoted
by the use of emmenagogues.   At the end
of three months she menstruated freely,
but with more than usual pain; which
was soon relieved by the use of opiates
and the warm pediluvium.   She now began to be more rational and agreeable in
her speech and behaviour, and would
civilly ask for her food and medicines;
and after five weeks continuance in the
above methods, she recovered the same
degree of reason she had possessed before
her illness, was well enough to return
home, and has not since experienced
any relapse.

CASE

CASE XXXV.

M. M. a very fenfible good kind of woman, fuffered much care and anxiety on account of a ceffation of the menfes, at a period when that event might reafonably be expected. The practitioner to whom fhe applied, rather fupported than fuppreffed the diftreffing notions which fhe entertained on this head; a regimen was propofed, and a medical plan determined upon: but having, from the alteration in her conftitution, unfortunately imbibed the moft melancholy ideas, and being prepoffeffed in the opinion that it would prove fatal, it operated with the worft effect on a mind too replete with fenfibility; in confequence of which fhe was continually terrifying herfelf with apprehenfions of the moft ferious nature, till by a continual courfe of folicitude, her mental faculties became impaired. As yet, however, fhe had fuffered but little interruption in her health, when fhe was fuddenly attacked with all the figns

of

of plethora, with fpafmodic affections of
various parts, dry cough, reftlefs nights,
frightful and extravagant dreams; with
inflammation in the eyes, heat, flufhings,
head-ach, ftupor, and dejection.

In this ftate of the cafe, an eminent
practitioner in town was applied to; and
as fhe had been accuftomed to copious
evacuations, very judicioufly directed her
to lofe fmall quantities of blood, her diet
to be moderated, and the bowels to be
kept open by proper food and medicine.
In this manner fhe proceeded for feveral
months, being always fubject at the ufual
periods of menftruation to profufe fweats,
violent heats, and pain in the lumbar region; at which time her reafon appeared
lefs impaired than ufual for the fpace of
two or three days, but afterwards the delirium returned, and continued fo till the
above period recurred, and produced the
fame effects. As the violence of the fymptoms rendered it neceffary at firft, fhe continued to lofe four or five ounces of blood
every month afterwards; but as her ftrength
apparently decreafed with the frequency of

L   this

this operation, and her mind was not relieved, it was protracted to longer periods;
fhe continued to take gentle laxatives, was
carefully watched and attended to; and
except fome nervous affections, which were
always obferved to be worfe at the cuftomary æra, remained for fome weeks tolerably well in bodily health, but on a fudden fhe was attacked with an immoderate
uterine flux; when reft, aftringents, and
anodynes were fuccefIively adminiftered.
She was greatly enfeebled by the hæmorrhage, and had fcarcely recovered a
moderate fhare of ftrength at the end of
fix weeks, when it returned again, and
the fame means of cure as were before
adopted, proved equally efficacious; and
the hæmorrhage ceafing, fuch medicines
as allay irritation and produce reft, with
a light nutritious diet, were prefcribed to
prevent a relapfe, and fhe remained pretty well till the return of the following
autumn, (a period of eleven weeks) when
fhe was feized with an intermittent complaint, and a return of the flux; and as
both obvioufly appeared to proceed from
                                    debility

debility and relaxation, the bark was judicioufly adminiftered, and had the defired
effect.

After this recovery, the patient regain-
ed her ftrength very faft; and being more
confiftent in her mind, at her own requeft,
and with the approbation of her relations,
returned into the country; but through the
officious care and obtrufion of a Female
Dabbler in Phyfic, who was too often
confulted in the management of her fex
at the ceffation of the menfes, fhe was induced to take repeated dofes of hiera
picra and aloetic pills, by whofe heating
qualities the piles and ftrangury were produced, with racking pains in the loins,
difficult refpiration, imbecility, and derangement of the intellects; pain in the
bowels, and a return of the uterine hæmorrhage.

In this emergency I was requefted to
prefcribe; and upon inquiry became acquainted with the above particulars. The
patient did not feem much debilitated by
the prefent difcharge; and as the ftate of
the pulfe evinced the propriety, I directed

four

four ounces of blood to be taken from
the arm, which, when cold, was covered
with a thin gluten, and the pulfe appeared
rather lowered and weakened by the operation. An emollient clyfter was adminiftered; and by a courfe of antiphlogiftic medicines, anodynes, reft, and a fparing
diet, the patient was in three weeks thoroughly recovered from the dangerous
ftate into which fhe had been precipitated
by the extreme ignorance of this Lady
Doctor. A period of life fo critically
important to the fex, as when the menfes
ceafe, deferves the confideration of the moft
judicious practitioner, and ought never to
be trifled with or fubmitted to the decifion of the inexperienced in either fex.

Having been informed that the patient,
a few years before this period, had been
fubject to fmall ulcers behind the ears,
and on fome parts of the head, difcharging
a humour which dried into a white cruft,
with pain in the eyes, and forenefs and
tumefaction of the eye-lids, which gradually difappeared foon after the commencement of the regular catamenia, and fhe
                                    had

had often complained of pains in the breafts
and other glandular parts, I advifed a feton
to be made between the fcapulæ, which being rejected, an iffue in the arm was propofed and acceded to. I recommended the
ftricteft attention to regimen and exercife,
and befought her moft earneftly to depre-
cate all fuch dangerous and pertinacious
advice, of which fhe had fo painfully
experienced the bad effects.

The alienation of mind which had been
perceived upon this laft attack, receded
with the fymptoms that had occafioned
it; and fhe continued tolerably well for a
year and a half afterwards, but was rather
inclined to plethora; when by remaining
too long at an affembly, fhe was feized
with rigors and chillnefs, to which fucceeded inflammation of the tonfils, attended with an eryfipetalous eruption upon the left fide of the neck and face, a
fpafmodic affection of the bowels, a naufea
and ficknefs of the ftomach, and a flight
flux from the uterine veffels; wandering
pains, conftriction of the breaft, difficulty
of breathing, inquietude, very little fleep,
hurry and confufion of thought, and much
incongruity

incongruity of action and behaviour. She was bled, had a blifter, and by the fame treatment as had been purfued on former occafions, was again reftored; has continued in good health for fome years paft, and ftill remains free from mania.

---

*CASE XXXVI.

THE late happy and providential efcape of his Majefty from the horrid attempt of affaffination by the hand of an infatuated maniac, appears in itfelf fufficient to determine all thofe under whofe care and protection fuch unfortunate perfons are placed, not to truft them too much to themfelves, or permit them to ramble at large. Many of thefe diforder-ed people may for fome time, nay even years, appear inoffenfive and harmlefs; yet from a ftrict and long acquaintance with maniacal patients, I am firmly of opinion that there can be no thorough

* Publifhed in the firft edition of this work in 1, 87, alluding to the affair of Margaret Nicholfon.

fecurity

fecurity or dependence at any time, in
any fituation, or under any circumftance,
to be placed in either their words or actions. As no perfon can determine how
momentarily their diforder may return or
increafe, it confequently behoves thofe who
have them under their command, to be
conftantly upon their guard ; nor fhould
their friends and relations be too hafty
in forming a judgment of their recovery,
as to the fafety of their return to their
accuftomed mode of life : for after recovering from a ftate of infanity, for fome
time the mind is as weak as the body,
after being afflicted with any violent
diforder.   And as in the one cafe the
patient cannot return to exercife and
diet as ufual in time of health, without
danger of a relapfe ; fo in the other he cannot return to his former objects, and avocations of life, without running the utmoft
rifque of his mind being again overfet and
deranged. A relapfe in this cafe is more to
be apprehended and guarded againft, than
in any other ; and it fhould never be forgotten that fuch convalefcents, either
from

from a temporary fenfation of joy, fudden prejudices, unaccountable averfions, an extravagance of fuperftitious notions, or any other caufe, may fuddenly have their mind put off its poife. Patients, therefore, under fuch circumftances, fhould be re-admitted into fociety with a particular degree of caution and circumfpection, as is evinced by numerous inftances recited in the public prints, as well as from many authors who have written on the fubject of infanity.

To corroborate thefe remarks from my own obfervation, I could adduce many inftances; but fhall at prefent felect only one, the melancholy effects of which are ftill painfully remembered by the furvivors of the worthy and refpectable family of the unfortunate lunatic. He held a commiffion in the army in the year 1748, and retained it upon half-pay till the time of his death, which happened in the year 1782. He was the eldeft fon of an ancient family in Cambridgefhire, and naturally of a morofe, arrogant, and imperious difpofition; whimfical, fly, and fufpicious;

fufpicious; but no very extraordinary fin-
gularities in his manner and behaviour
became remarkable till the autumn of
1776, when he was fuddenly feized with
an hypochondriacal affection, attended
with vehement motions of the body, fear,
fufpicion, impatience, and violent perturbations of mind, which at length fettled
into a deep melancholy; but he did not
attempt any violence either to himfelf or
others. After proper attention and medical affiftance, he was fuppofed to have
intirely recovered from this diforder, and
thought in every refpect to be as well as
ufual, when on a fudden he became poffeffed of the moft abfurd and ftrange fancies, fufpicions, and averfions. He was
reftlefs, timid, irrefolute, and weak in his
judgment, which was lefs obfervable, as
he was never remarkable for the moft
lively feelings, or the greateft brilliancy of
imagination. He fpoke and acted in an
unufually ridiculous manner.

He was fent to a houfe appropriate for
the reception of infane perfons, in the vicinity of the metropolis; in which fituation

tion he had not continued many weeks, before his mother and a near relation, impelled by the natural attachment of affinity, went to pay him a visit. He seemed exceedingly glad to see them, and used the most specious and plausible arguments and pretences, with all that subdolous art and cunning so inseparably attached to lunacy; by which seemingly consistent behaviour he so far imposed upon their credulity, as to cause them to believe him in his right senses. Throughout a long conversation he appeared so perfectly cool, consistent, and rational, as determined them to grant him his enlargement. Accordingly the next day he was liberated, and sent home, where for about a week his behaviour was such as to justify their conduct; but getting up one morning earlier than usual, and coming home wet and dirty, after a frantic excursion of some miles, he abruptly walked into the parlour where his mother was sitting at work, who seeing him in this dishabille, gently reproved him, expressed some concern at his appearance, and requested quefted him to make himfelf clean, and get his breakfaft; when, fhocking to relate! the maniac inftantly without the leaft hefitation, and before fhe could get any affiftance, fnatched up a poker which was ftanding in the fire-place, and dafhed her brains out upon the floor. The noife and buftle brought in the fervants; but *the maniac parricide* offering no farther violence, was foon difarmed of the fatal weapon, and fecured. He did not attempt to efcape, nor did he appear then, or at any other time after, to feel the leaft compunction or remorfe for this dreadful tranfaction. Soon after which he was committed to my care, and in about three years afterwards died of an hydrops pectoris, in the fifty-firft year of his age.

Not diffimilar in point of miftaken affection, will be found the following paragraph, taken from a public print, fo late as the 23d of April 1797. A letter from Haddington in Scotland, fays, " A me-
" lancholy event has happened in that
" neighbourhood. Major Kenlock, the
" brother of Sir Francis Kenlock, of Gel-
" maton,

" maton, was obferved for fome time to
" be deranged in his fenfes.   His brother
" Sir Francis, whofe affe&tion would not
" fuffer the neceffary means of reftraint
" to be ufed, trufted he fhould be able
" to calm his phrenfy, and to reftore him
" to reafon, or at leaft to keep the domef-
" tic calamity from becoming a public
" topic.   The major was extremely vio-
" lent, went about the houfe and grounds
" armed with a blunderbufs and piftols,
" threatening with death any perfon who
" ftopped his way. On Tuefday night
" laft, Sir Francis prevailed upon him to
" retire to his apartment; but at three
" o'clock in the morning, when he thought
" the family were in bed, he quitted his
" room, and went down ftairs, to fally out
" of the houfe, but was met by Sir Francis,
" who endeavoured to perfuade him to
" return.   The major immediately drew
" a piftol and fhot him. He languifhed
" till Thurfday afternoon, when he died!

    " The maniac (now Sir Archibald
" Kenlock, as he fucceeds to the title and
" eftate) was confined in Haddington gaol,
                                " to

" to take his trial for the horrid deed;
" when it appeared before the high court
" of justiciary at Edinburgh, that while in
" the West-Indies he had been seized with
" a fever; from which time he was never
" considered as possessed of a *sound mind,*
" but was subject to melancholy, with fits
" of jealousy; and that at the time this
" unhappy transaction was committed, he
" was in the most lamentable state of
" derangement. He was sentenced to
" be confined the rest of his life."

CASE XXXVII.

I Am indebted for the subsequent case
to the communication of an obliging cor-
respondent, on whose authority I can
safely rely. In the beginning of the month
of February 1777, a poor man was bitten
in the calf of the leg by a dog that was
mad. He was immediately bled, blistered
upon the part, dipped in the salt water,
and took a nostrum of some celebrity in
the

the place where he lived: after which he was
directed to drink cold water till he threw
it up again by vomiting. Dry cupping,
mercury, fcarifications, the warm bath,
and fea bathing were alternately ufed. His
diet was ordered to be light and laxative;
and he underwent a courfe of antifpafmodic medicines. The wound was entirely
healed, and a cicatrix formed in the part.
However, about the eighth of March following, being more than a month from the
time the accident happened, he began to
complain of pricking fhooting fenfations, attended with heat, and wandering pains like
thofe which attend rheumatifm, in all his
joints and limbs; the healed parts fwelled,
inflamed, and difcharged an ichorous humour; he became penfive, tremulous,
watchful, prone to anger; his face was
pale and contracted; he was drowfy; had
a drynefs and heat in the fauces; foulnefs
of the tongue, foetid breath, and his fleep
was difturbed with convulfive agitations;
fymptoms which were confidered by the
furgeon who attended him as the indications of incipient hydrophobia. He complained

plained of ſtricture and weight acroſs the
breaſt ; tingling in his ears ; loſs of hearing ; was weary, inactive, and torpid ;
vomited bile of an eruginous colour ;
the ſtomach was extended, and a conſtric-
tion of the gullet was evident. The *pavor
aquæ*, or dread of water, ſoon ſucceeded ;
and every attempt to ſwallow excited the
moſt dreadful convulſions, with the in-
tenſeſt horror, fear, and averſion at the
ſight of it. At intervals he was ſtill capable of making rational anſwers, and entirely free from the convulſive paroxyſm,
which returned upon every freſh attempt
to ſwallow, or even to taſte any thing that
was liquid : and although he was parched
and burnt with an eager deſire to drink,
yet no ſooner did any liquid touch the tip
of his tongue, than he was inſtantly ſeized
with the moſt terrible ſtricture of the jaws,
ſucceeded by univerſal convulſions of the
whole frame, that intirely deprived him of
his ſenſes. There was a moſt remarkable
dilatation of the pupils, and he could not
ſee. The larynx was externally ſwelled,
                              and

and fuddenly rofe and fell. He had frequent regurgitation of the ftomach; his eyes had been bright and fierce, and his afpect wild and threatening; but on the third day from his firft attack, his eyes became more dull and opaque. The fpafms returned at fhorter intervals; a conftant delirium, with deep fighing, took place; and on the evening of the third day, nature being quite worn out and exhaufted, the unhappy fufferer refigned his breath without a ftruggle!

During the progrefs of the complaint, he was never obferved to have any unufual flow of faliva, nor did he ever fnarl or bark like a dog, or endeavour to bite any one about him. Cupping with and without fcarification, mercury, the warm bath, &c. all proved ineffectual in this and two other cafes which fell under my obfervation, and the unfortunate fufferers died of the complaint; the one in about feven weeks after the accident, and the other in lefs time. It is therefore highly neceffary, and of the firft importance to every per-

fon

fon who is fo unfortunate as to be bitten by a mad dog, or other animal fo affected, to fubmit to the *total excifion* of the wounded parts, as this method is *alone* to be depended upon for the prevention of the complaint. It is inconteftibly proved, that no confidence whatever can be placed in any of the boafted medicines for this purpofe; either Palmarius's powder, mercurial friction, fomentations of fea falt and vinegar, the pulvis antilyffus, tonquinefa, the Ormfkirk medicine, the famous pewter preparation, or any other pretended fpecific; all of which in their turns have been found totally inadequate to oppofe the evil they were intended to defeat. Mufk and the warm bath, fea bathing, antifpafmodics, and even cauftics themfelves, have likewife been too often ufed without fuccefs: therefore, *timely excifion and ablution* with water of the bitten parts, feem to be the only and truly efficacious remedies. For to flatter perfons with fecurity from other methods, is only to deceive them in a matter of the utmoft confequence, which in the end proves fatal

M   by

by the occurrence of that melancholy cataſtrophe—death! through the medium of an incurable and raging madneſs.

The third volume of the Memoirs of the Medical Society of London, furniſhes us with the following remarks; being a letter from Dr. White of St. Edmunds-bury to Dr. Lettſom.

" In the laſt nine months, this part of " the country has been terribly infeſted " with mad dogs; during which time it " has been my misfortune to be applied to " by ſeveral perſons who have been bitten, " and as I myſelf have been, *'anxious and* " *trembling for the birth of fate.'* Seven " of theſe miſerable objects were bitten " by dogs quite unprovoked, and with " every appearance of raging madneſs. " Three did not apply till the third day, " two on the ſecond day, and two in a few " hours after the accident. Three others " have alſo been with me for advice, who " were bitten by a cow that had the hy-" drophobia. All of theſe, except two, " had the injured parts wholly diſſected " out, the wounds well waſhed firſt with " cold

" cold and then with warm water, and
" the furface touched with lunar cauftic.
" One of the excepted two was bitten
" about eight months ago in the palm and
" the back of the hand; in which cafe
" fuch of the wounded part as could be
" with fafety, was removed, and the pro-
" cefs of ablution continued for near two
" hours; nothing having been done exter-
" nally till the day on which I was con-
" fulted, which was the third from the
" accident. This perfon is in her full
" health and fpirits: and in the other
" inftance, as the tooth of the cow had
" penetrated the end of the finger, through
" the nail, I thought myfelf warranted to
" deprive the patient of the firft joint.
" It is now five months or more fince I
" was confulted about a foal which had
" been bitten by a mad dog, through the
" wing of the left noftril. The wounded
" part was much torn; I ordered it to be
" cut out, and no other means were ufed.
" The animal is at this time perfectly well,
" and is a ufeful horfe. A cow and two
" pigs were bitten by the fame dog; to

M 2   " which

" which external remedies only were ufed:
" they all died mad within the month.
" Similar collateral circumftances occur-
" red to prove that the dog was mad. Out
" of the feven inftances before-mentioned,
" on which external means only , were
" employed, two perfons on whom *exci-*
" *fion* and *ablution* had not been per-
" formed, and to whom medicines of falfe
" repute had been given, fell victims to
" their credulity.

" This brief detail of accidents that
" have lately fallen under my care, to-
" gether with the remembrance of four
" cafes of hydrophobia which I have been
" called to in the courfe of my practice,
" have given rife to the following fug-
" geftions:

" That the virus may be extirpated
" by *excifion* many days after the acci-
" dent.

" That the firft fenfible mark of its ac-
" tion is pain in the injured part.

" That the confequent fymptoms and
" fenfations have a much nearer relation
" to fpafm than to inflammation.

" That

" That the lymphatic fyftem is not
" affected in the manner that it is by the
" infertion of the variolous, or any other
" infectious matter, fuppofed to be car-
" ried into the habit by abforption.

" Admitting thefe premifes, is it not
" probable," fays our author, " that the
" virus lays dormant till the previous
" fymptom (pain) comes on in the bitten
" part ? Might not excifion and ablution,
" therefore, afford relief at that period?
" May not the future progreffive fymp-
" toms be produced by irregular excite-
" ment on the nervous fyftem only?

" Is it abfolutely impoffible to give re-
" lief by *excifion*, &c. when the patient is
" affected with hydrophobia ?

" As the virus is more commonly, per-
" haps folely generated in animals that
" never perfpire, will the cow, or any
" other kind of creature, not fubject to
" that peculiarity, produce, or in the hy-
" drophobic ftate communicate, the dif-
" eafe ?"

CASE

CASE XXXVIII.

AFTER long and fevere fits of an intermittent fever, a tradefman in Jewry-
ftreet, Weftminfter, aged thirty-four, applied to me on the 22nd of October 1784.
He informed me that about fix weeks before, an abfcefs had formed in his leg,
which fuppurated, and after a copious difcharge for the fpace of three weeks, had
fuddenly dried up; fince which he had
been fubject to great anxiety of mind, with
a fenfe of weight and coldnefs in both his
legs, and pain in the ftomach, wind, noifes
and rumblings in the bowels, and palpitations of the heart. His appetite was depraved; he had tenfion in the left hypochondrium, with conftant flight pains; his
breath had been extremely offenfive; his
fpirits were depreffed; and his hearing
was not fo good as before. He alfo complained of a head-ach, in a fingle fmall fpot
over the left orbit, as if a nail was driven
into the head; of finging in his ears, debility, thirft, a frequent dimnefs of fight;
the

the pulſe was weak and irregular; the pupils of his eyes were much dilated, but more particularly the left; he had horrid notions of ſupernatural agents, and his aſpect was wild and unſettled. He had been coſtive; and informed me that his urine had in general been colourleſs, forming no cloud, and depoſiting no ſediment; that he was naturally timid, irreſolute, prone to ſudden and exceſſive paſſions of the mind, and for ſome time paſt had paid too ſerious an attention to the noiſy and dangerous harangues of a methodiſt preacher in the neighbourhood where he reſided, which had induced him frequently to conclude in his own mind that he had loſt all chance of ſalvation, and the favour of his Maker; the thought of which often overwhelmed him with horror and dread, and threw him into tremblings and ſpaſms; and as his habit appeared much debilitated and weakened, I adviſed him to uſe cold bathing, and a more liberal diet, to encourage every method of promoting cheerfulneſs and ſerenity of mind, and entirely to relinquiſh

the

the falfe and mifchievous doctrines of his
enthufiaftic preceptor; to have an iffue
made in the leg, where the abfcefs had
formed, and was now dried up; and with
a view to ftrengthen and brace the fyftem,
I recommended him to a courfe of the
Pyrmont waters. After this I heard nothing more of him till I received an order
to take him into my houfe as a lunatic,
which was on the 13th of December following.

When committed to my care, he
laboured under violent depreffion of
mind, complained of the moft uncom-
fortable bodily feelings and mental per-
plexities; and every trifling occurrence
produced an object of inquietude and
vexation; he was coftive, and ftill complained of the fame pain in his head as
when I firft faw him, with ftupor, tumefaction of the eye-lids, and flight inflammation of the eyes. The warm pediluvium, and a feton between the fhoulders
in the direction of the fpine, were ordered. The camphorated mixture was adminiftered thrice in twenty-four hours,
and

and his body kept open and cool by a proper regimen, and the ol. ricini: which practice (with the addition only of fumigations of rosemary, camphor, and vinegar, to his head and face, every night and morning) was sanctioned by the concurrence of an eminent physician who was consulted in conjunction with myself, at the particular desire of his friends; and in about eight weeks he was so thoroughly recovered in his intellects, as to become consistently conversant and sociable. As his complaints were now entirely of the nervous and relaxed kind, he was directed to go to Bath, where he found much relief, and was so entirely recovered as to be able to return to his business, in which he has ever since continued without the least mental or corporeal complaint.

As this patient's insanity, as well as that of which I shall next treat, happened after a fever, I shall here quote the opinion of the celeberated Hoffman, who mentions insanity of every species as frequently occurring after fevers, and especially so if

protracted

protracted to a great length; and accounts for this circumstance from the dissipation of the animal spirits by the violent and long-continued heat and watching, by a defect in their secretion, in consequence of an injury done to the fibrous texture of the brain, and of the whole animal system.

CASE XXXIX.

M. O. was of a thin hectic constitution, and had for many years laboured under a troublesome pulmonary cough. When I first visited her, the pulse was remarkably quick and sharp; her eyes were in continual motion, and her face was of an unusually florid hue: she possessed the advantages of a polite education, and had always been peculiarly sensible, brisk, and lively, till soon after her recovery from a long protracted and acute fever: she then became torpid, and lost in an unthinking joyless inactivity; from which, if at any time

time fhe recovered, or was roufed, delirium, fear, terror, and agitation of fpirits fupervened, until fhe reverted into her
former torpidity; and in one of thofe intervals of horror fhe had even attempted
to put an end to her life, but was happily
prevented. Gentle opiates, with a variety of balfamic medicines, had been given
to palliate her cough, which was flight,
fhort, frequent, and without expectoration. The warm pediluvium was ufed
every evening at bed-time, a perpetual
blifter opened between her fhoulders, and
the camphorated mixture given three
or four times a day; but thefe means
proving ineffectual, a preparation of milli-
pedes with the oxymel of fquills, the balfamic pills, and an infufion of madder
root, were next tried. Change of air, exercife, and the Briftol waters, were prefcribed, but to no kind of purpofe; for
the unfortunate patient grew worfe, and
in three months time, without ever recovering the leaft ray of intellectual light,
fhe expired.

CASE

CASE XL.

ABOUT five years ago, M. S. about eighteen years of age, of a ruddy fanguine complexion, and till then very healthy, fuddenly complained of a ftrangulation of the fauces, humour and hardnefs in the neck, wandering pains, laffitude, conftriction of the thorax, and fpafms of the maxillæ, with frequent fainting and exceffive menftruation. A practitioner of eminence was called to her affiftance, and in a few days fhe recovered; but from that period her mind became very much hurried and difturbed; there was an unufual fiercenefs in her eyes, and the prevailing fymptom was anger, which often exhibited itfelf in fuch violent and groundlefs rage that it became abfolutely neceffary to confine her. She was naturally meek and gentle, of an amiable difpofition, and not in the leaft difpofed to be irritable; but was now become morofe, peevifh, contentious, and determined on mifchief of the moft violent and defperate nature; fhe replied

in

in an impetuous tone of anger to every one who accofted, or converfed with her; flept but little, and perfpired lefs; fometimes fhe raved aloud, and at others fpit at and endeavoured to bite thofe about her; foamed at the mouth with anger, and whiftled, fung, fhouted, or fwore alternately.

In this precife ftate I found her on the 12th of March 1784. The tunica albuginea of the eyes was ftreaked with red, her countenance fixed, her head hot, the pulfe quick and full, her tongue white and furred; there was a fordes upon her teeth and lips, the eye-lids were puffed and tumefied, and a kind of infpiffated mucus abounded about the mouth, throat, and trachea, which was much increafed by the vehemence of her actions and geftures. Befides thefe fymptoms, the fkin was dry and harfh; her features had rather a greafy appearance; fhe had no appetite; her breath was hot and fœtid; fhe had frequent eructations; her refpiration was difficult by paroxyfms attended with rigor, reftleffnefs, and watching. She had had but

but one ftool for the three laft days, which was remarkably high coloured, bilious, and offenfive; fhe often gnafhed her teeth; paffed her urine involuntarily; groaned, yawned, and fighed. Upon opening a vein in the arm, four ounces of blood had been taken away; when the pulfe flagged and funk from eighty to below fixty ftrokes in a minute; and a fyncope coming on, the orifice was clofed. The blood, when cold, was covered with a thin cake of gluten. The evening after the operation, the antimon. tartar. was prefcribed in fuch dofes as to puke her gently, which was repeated every twelve hours, and the body kept open by an emollient laxative clyfter. A feton was made between the fhoulders in the direction of the fpine, and an emulfion given with the kali tartarifat. to keep her bowels in a cool and lax ftate; in the intermediate fpace, the camphorated mixture to abate the increafed ofcillatory contractions of the veffels, was prefcribed. Fomentations of poppy heads, and chamomile flowers, were applied to the feet and legs, and the fymptoms gradually

dually abating, in little more than a fortnight fhe became compofed and rational;
and in lefs than a month was capable
of correfponding by letter with a lady of
her acquaintance, to whofe houfe, after
recruiting her ftrength with a courfe of
bark, aromatic bitters, and Bath waters,
fhe made a vifit; and eftablifhed in a good
ftate of health, foon afterwards, with the
confent and approbation of her friends,
fhe entered into the matrimonial ftate, by
which all her wifhes were accomplifhed,
and her happinefs was complete.

CASE XLI.

THE Rev. J. R. of relaxed fibres and
fcorbutic temperament from his infancy,
was naturally of a cheerful turn of temper, and of an open generous difpofition,
till he fuftained the preffure of a particular afflicttion, which occurred to a very
near relation, when he fell a victim to the
moft anxious and diftrefsful feelings,
by which means his body was gradually
weakened,

weakened, and his reafon fo much impaired, that he had always the moft harraffing
and difmal train of ideas continually before him, and was almoft ever under the
influence of defpair, grief, and lamen-
tation, in which ftate he had continued
many months; and in that time undergone the whole routine of nervous
medicines—with antimonials, purges, fe-
gapenum, fteel, kali tart. hellebore, &c.
but his imagination was ftill difturbed,
and his reafon perverted.

In April 1784, I was confulted on his
fituation; diftrefs and melancholy were
deeply engraven on his features, and internal anguifh and horror had overwhelmed his mind; his face was pale and
fallow; his hands and feet were puffed
and red; he often hiccoughed, and fpoke
with a peculiar hollow voice; the pulfe
was hard; and he had frequently a palpitation of the heart. The refpiration was
deep and flow; he was wakeful in the
extreme; and his fkin felt dry, hard, and
fqualid; he had not perfpired in the
leaft; and when he fpoke, there was a
                                    particular

particular tremor of the tongue; he had no fever; and there was a vifible wafting of his flefh.   Which ftate of body was occafioned by the exceffive diftrefs of his mind; the agonizing influence of which afforded me very little reafon to hope, or even imagine, that the ufual means of cure would prove efficient.   In this refpect I was truly forry to find myfelf not in the leaft difappointed; for after he had been under my care a confiderable length of time, and the warm bath, pediluvium, electricity, emetics, cupping with and without fcarification, cephalic fteams, mufk, camphor, a feton, iffues, blifters, æther, various cephalics and antifpafmodic remedies had refpectively been tried, every hope and expectation of relief vanifhed, and the unfortunate patient was configned to permanent care and confinement, as the *dernier refort* of his afflicted family.

CASE

CASE XLII.

Among the caufes of infanity, it is
ufual to attribute the complaint to fome
affeƈtion of the brain, its veffels or membranes; fuch as diftention, preternatural
enlargement, malformations, indurations,
&c. and the remote caufes are generally
confidered to be too intenfe an application
of the mind to ftudy, bufinefs, or fchemes
of any kind, which require an unremitting
attention or uncommon exertion of genius; to fudden, violent, or habitual paffions of various kinds, &c.; and here our
difquifitions generally terminate.   I am of
opinion, that were we oftener to extend
our inquiries by minutely tracing them
back in a genealogical line to the proge-
nitors of thofe labouring under confirmed
mania, we fhould more generally adopt
the opinion that the much greater number
of mankind, who become infane from any
particular change in conftitution, have an
hereditary pre-difpofition to madnefs; nor
is this mere hypothefis and conjeƈture; the
faƈt

fact being founded on the folid bafis of the
moft extenfive obfervation and experience.
Of the greateft number of maniacal patients that have been placed under my
care in the courfe of more than thirty
years practice, I have been able to trace
an hereditary pretenfion to this diforder
in by much the major part of them : to
maintain this pofition, on the bafis of
found fact, I have in moft cafes preferved
an exact courfe of genealogy in regular
lineal defcent home to the deftined object.

A gentleman of large commercial concerns in the city, after much clofe and intenfe ftudy, was fuddenly feized with a pain
in the calf of his leg, with palpitation about
the navel ; at the fame time he complained
of throbbing in his head and temples, and
had fome flight degree of febrile heat.
Thefe fymptoms were at firft attributed to
obftructed perfpiration from the effects of
cold ; and as the moft probable means of
relief, bleeding was prefcribed, and afterwards the reguline preparations at proper
diftances, and the faline draughts were
given in the intermediate fpaces; but it
foon after appeared that the functions of his

mind

mind had been injured by too clofe an application to bufinefs, and he now prefented a difpofition of mind entirely repugnant to his natural feelings; he railed at and quarrelled with all who approached him, and fhewed an uncommon hatred to particular perfons who had never injured him; had but little fleep; fpoke with furlinefs and ill-nature; fufpected every one of finifter views and nefarious intentions, and even thofe in whom he ufed to place an unlimited confidence in concerns of the greateft importance. In his countenance was marked the ftrongeft traits of fufpicion and rancour; he feemed ftudioufly anxious to avoid all converfation; and the very appearance of his own fpecies filled him with fcorn, hatred, and difguft. If fpoken to, he would frown and look with contumely, or turn away with filent contempt, or mutter malice and diflike. And to borrow the allufion of Shakefpeare, " his wits feemed loft and " drowned in his calamities."

In this truly fad and mifanthropic ftate of mind, he was entrufted to the care of a phy-

fician,

fician, as much diftinguifhed for his honor
and integrity, as for his fuperiority of profeffional fkill and experience. Management was allowed to be of the firft confequence in this cafe, to which was added
fuch medical treatment as the various indications rendered neceffary. After every
experiment of this nature had been tried
for more than three months, the former
was adopted, and the latter entirely
laid afide; at which period the patient
was entrufted to my care. His appetite
was natural, but he would never eat any
thing unlefs it was left in his room; and
then he perfifted in its having been taken
from him by ftealth; his features were
contracted, his eye-lids puffed and fwelled,
the pupils much dilated, and his eyes
very ftrongly indicated the ftate of his
mind; he was coftive, and never perfpired; his pulfe was weak, foft, and un-
dulating; his fkin pale, harfh, and fallow; and he appeared much emaciated.
After trying a feton, cupping, the warm
bath, cephalic fteams, camphor, mufk,
and emetics, to no purpofe, and every
medical

medical effort had been relinquifhed for
more than three months, the patient on a
fudden recovered his fenfe and reafon, and
continuing in this ftate for a confiderable
time, was permitted to return home ;
but had not long renewed his application
to bufinefs, before he unfortunately reverted into his former ftate of infanity,
and continued fo for nearly the fame
fpace of time as before, and then as fuddenly recovered. Thefe infane and lucid
intervals periodically fucceeded each other
during fome years. On making proper inquiry I difcovered that the grandfather of
this unfortunate gentleman was afflicted
with a fimilar fpecies of infanity for a confiderable time before his death.

CASE XLIII.

J. C. of Buxted, in Suffex, aged about
fix-and-thirty, of a fanguine habit and
fcorbutic temperament, had been afflicted
with lunacy for many months. He had
taken many vomits, been bliftered, and
ufed

ufed feveral methods for relief without fuccefs.   January 9th, 1785, he was fent to
my houfe, in a condition nearly approaching to raving madnefs.   His appetite was
voracious, his breath offenfive, he was coftive, and had a particular difficulty of deglutition ; his eyes were bright, fiery, protuberant, and wild ; the lids tumefied, and
the pupils much diftended ; he often raifed
his hand to his head, and complained of
pain in his forehead ; the pulfe was ftrong,
and his countenance bloated ; but he had
little or no heat. The right hypochondrium
was fwelled and tenfe, and his breathing was
rather difficult ; he had been fubject to the
hæmorrhoids before he was attacked with
mania, but they had entirely difappeared
for many months.   He had flept but little,
and his fkin was dry and harfh ; the urine
was generally high coloured, and depofited a copious red fediment of the nature
of bran ; with fudden tranfitions of mind,
and rapid flights of imagination ; was
noify, furious, audacious, impetuous, or
mifchievous ; would laugh, fing, rave, or
talk vociferoufly, in the fame inftant, with
quick

quick tranfitions from one fubject to another, as different images and fancies
occurred to his difturbed mind.   Sixteen
ounces of blood were taken from him on
the third day after his coming to me,
which, when cold, indicated fome degree
of inflammation; and as he appeared not
in the leaft weakened by its lofs, and continued nearly as furious as before, on the
fourth morning after the firft operation it
was repeated in fufficient quantity to produce deliquium, which in this and every
other cafe where phlebotomy is neceffary,
ufque ad deliquium animi, it is obfervable is
moft fpeedily effected by keeping the patient
in an erect pofition during the hæmorrhage.
The fame evening he took an antimonial
vomit, which brought away a great quantity of dark, bilious, vifcid matter.   For his
coftivenefs, the ol. ricini folut. and the foda
phofphorata, were occafionally adminiftered, and the warm pediluvium was ufed
every evening. The camphorated mixture
with nitre was given him every fix hours.
His head was fhaved, and frequently embrocated with fp. rorifmarini aq diftill. and
vinegar,

vinegar, in due proportions. A liniment of
camphor and oil was applied to the right
hypochondrium twice a day.   This courfe
was continued with little variation, and
a due regard to his regimen, for feveral weeks, without any apparent benefit.
To the difficulty of fwallowing was now
added oppreffion of breathing, which was
always relieved for a few days by an emetic; and now the pil. fcillæ, with calomel,
were advifed, alfo a feton in the neck in
the direction of the fpine, and half an
ounce of kali tartarifat. in weak broth,
every third morning, which feldom failed
of procuring him two or three motions.
The feton difcharging in a very copious
manner, in lefs than a month his flights,
ravings, anxieties, and vociferations were
moderated ; but he was yet very incoherent, although at times more intelligent
than he had been fince the commencement
of his diforder, when he would attend to
what was faid to him, and fometimes make
pertinent replies.   On a fudden the hæmorrhoids re-appeared, and difcharged
profufely, and at the fame time his fanity
returned,

returned, and continued in its full force. Gently cooling medicines were adminif-tered to keep the body open, which, to-gether with the ufe of emollient liniments and fomentations, foon relieved the hæ-morrhoidal complaint ; after which he underwent a courfe of alteratives and anti-fcorbutics, and at the beginning of July re-turned home to his family, fo well reftored in body and mind, that I have not heard he has fince experienced the leaft relapfe.

CASE XLIV.

Mr. J. F. an eminent attorney in Lon-don, confulted me concerning his wife, in the month of December 1787. She had borne feveral children, and was in her forty-fifth year, naturally of a fufceptible, lively, and amiable difpofition, but at inter-vals had long been fubject to a melancholic fpecies of infanity, for which fhe had taken the advice of a phyfician, but to no effect. Her anguifh of mind was tormenting to

an

an extreme degree, and her feelings exquifitely fevere. She was fo much fubject to flatulencies of the ftomach and
vifcera, as fometimes occafioned a tumour
in the abdomen, of a globular form, as large
as a child's head, attended with fuch great
pain and tenfion, that made her cry out
as if fhe were in labour, which in her
depraved ftate of mind fhe would often
affert to be the cafe, requiring immediate
affiftance to receive and fave the child.
This fymptom never failed of palliation
from a warm ftomach purge of a carminative quality, and proper topical applications. It was obfervable, that when fhe
fuffered moft pain from this flatulent diftenfion of the abdomen, her intellects were
much clearer than at any other period
of her diforder; and upon the remiffion
of the complaint, fhe never failed to declare pofitively that fhe had been delivered
of a child, about which, however, fhe
never expreffed any great folicitude, nor
maternal tendernefs. An entire ceffation
of the menfes had taken place prior to
her becoming my patient. The pulfe
was

was in general hard and quick, her eyes were heavy and opaque, and the voice low, dull, and plaintive. I ordered fix ounces of blood to be taken from her arm, and an aperient and carminative electuary to be occasionally adminiftered, to keep her bowels in an undifturbed regularly aperient ftate. Her nights were rendered tolerably calm and compofed by means of the mift. camphor. She had a perpetual blifter: and the warm pediluvium was ufed every night at bed-time. The fp. æth. vitriol was given her in fmall quantities, in draughts of fimple peppermint water, every forenoon at eleven, and afternoon at five o'clock. After continuing in this mode of treatment fomething more than three months, fhe was thought well enough to be removed to her own houfe, where fhe foon experienced a relapfe, and after much viciffitude of diforder, died of a cholera morbus in about twelve months after her removal.

CASE

CASE XLV.

AMONGST all the active substances taken into the system, that immediately affect the circulation, and produce a change in the constitution, perhaps mercury demands the first place in our consideration; and in all the remote causes imputed to the use or abuse of this singularly powerful mineral, it may with propriety be often considered as a principle, which will obviously appear from the subsequent cases.

Carried away by the impulse of the passions, at a time of life when rational conduct and found judgment seldom preponderate, a young gentleman of a thin habit and slender constitution, found it necessary to apply to a surgeon of his acquaintance in town, who treated him in a manner suitable to his disorder. After six weeks, from irregularity in drinking, and a life of gaiety and dissipation, some symptoms of his complaint still remained, and he was suddenly attacked with an ulceration

of

of the tonfils, and other affections, which left
but little doubt of the blood being tainted
with the venereal virus, fo as to render it
neceffary to have recourfe to mercurial
alteratives, with a decoction of the woods;
but although, contrary to his ufual cuftom, he continued tolerably regular in this
courfe, he found himfelf in no one refpect
better, and was therefore advifed to
ftronger mercurial preparations, till his
complaints being apparently relieved, he
was induced to difcontinue his medicines,
and contrary to the advice of his furgeon,
to try the cold bath, which he had only
ufed twice, when he complained of great
pain in his head and cheft, with much
anxiety and inquietude, with a fenfation
of heat under the fternum, fucceeded by
vomiting, an obftinate conftipation, and a
remitting fever, the acerbations of which
returned once in twelve hours. From all
thefe fymptoms, by means of judicious
treatment, in lefs than a fortnight he was
entirely exempt, but complained of fome
fmall eruptions of a petechial appearance,
withinfide his mouth, and his fenfes became
much

much deranged. A folution of the fub-
limate was prefcribed for him twice a
day, with a proper gargle for his mouth;
he was ordered a light nourifhing diet,
with the ufe of the warm bath; but after
fome confiderable time, when there was
every reafon to fuppofe that the primary
diforder was removed, and no relapfe had
occurred to fhew the contrary, and every
care and precaution had been ufed by his
friends (who dreaded the impending evil)
to prevent it, he grew melancholy, ftupid,
and inactive, was reduced to the mental
weaknefs of a child, and dwindled into a
confirmed idiotifm, in which pitiable ftate

" Immured and buried in perpetual floth,
" The gloomy flumber of the vacant foul,"

he has continued for more than ten
years, and from which there is now
not the leaft probability that he will
ever emerge.

CASE

CASE XLVI.

W. D. of a robuft habit of body, and accuftomed to active life, through keeping late hours, exceffive drinking, and intemperately indulging in diffipation, in the forty-fixth year of his age contracted a diforder, for the relief of which it was deemed neceffary he fhould get advice in London, when the medicines moft fuitable to his cafe were adminiftered, and in a few weeks he was pronounced to be perfectly recovered. In about a month afterwards he fuddenly complained of heat, fever, head-ach, exceffive deafnefs, ulceration in the throat, and obftructed deglutition. At which crifis he returned to the metropolis, and went through a regular mercurial courfe, with the decoct. farfaparil. comp. This he continued for fix weeks, when (it being in the winter feafon) the weather became uncommonly cold, and he imprudently ftaying out to a very late hour; an obftructed perfpiration was the confequence, and a fenfe of coldnefs, with fhivering, which

which was fucceeded by naufea, vomiting,
thirft, anxiety, and comatous affections,
which were removed by epifpaftics and
the antiphlogiftic treatment. But there
remained an unufual ftupidity, and it was
obvious to all his friends, that the functions of his mind were confiderably impaired; he frequently complained of an
internal pain and weight in the left hypochondrium, extreme languor, difficult refpiration, giddinefs, and head-ach. His friends
confulted a phyfician in London, who
pronounced his malady to be an incipient madnefs. This prognoftication was
literally true; for notwithftanding the
moft approved methods adopted to prevent it, his mind became agitated with
various ill-forted ideas, and abfurd chime-
rical notions. The animal fpirits were
fubject to irregular fluctuations, and a
confirmed mania occurred. He alternately raved aloud, was turbulent, ungovernable, and outrageous; fometimes
cheerful and merry, and at others ftupid,
mufing, and melancholy. He would fit

o   for

for hours in evident pain, with his hand
to his forehead.   An eruption of a vesi-
cular nature appeared on his skin, accompanied with some pustules on the inside
of his mouth.   After this appearance it
was observed that he much seldomer lifted
his hand to his head. On the 25th of Auguft 1782, he was recommended to my
care, when I found an abscess had formed
on the tibia of the left leg, and terminated
in a large phagedenic ulcer.   I ordered a
feton to be paffed between the shoulders,
in the direction of the spine, the warm
pediluvium, and a solution of the subli-
mate and camphor; which being continued about six weeks, the delirious affection abated, the ulcer healed, and the eruption difappeared. To the ulcer was applied
the ung. hydragy. nitrat. but upon a dif-
continuance of the solution, in less than a
month after re-appeared in an accumulated
degree, when his mind seemed to be more
deranged than ever.   On repeating thefe
medicines, the mental and corporeal symptoms were for a time palliated, but soon
recurred;

recurred; fince which time his intellects have continued in a very confufed and difordered ftate, without any hopes of recovery.

―――――――

CASE XLVII.

J. T. a young man of family and for-tune, flender conftitution, and fcorbutic habit, in the year 1787, contracted a ve-nereal complaint, and put himfelf under the care of a furgeon, who adminiftered mercury and ftrong purges fo profufely, as to aggravate rather than relieve his dif-order. Several other remedies being in-ternally and externally applied, without producing the expected relief, falivation was deemed indifpenfably neceffary. This was accordingly put in practice, and a courfe of mercurial alteratives fucceed-ed. Ulcerations in the fauces, ton-fils, and throat, ftill remained. At this crifis he accidentally received a fall from a horfe, and fprained his ankle; as a remedy for which he was advifed to im-

merfe

merfe the leg in cold water, which he
had not often repeated before he experienced a total lofs of ftrength, fucceeded by inactivity, anxiety, difquietude of
mind, and a general derangement of idea,
fo that his words were fpoken without
either order or coherence; he fwallowed
with difficulty and pain; the tafte was impaired; and his voice was feeble and indiftinctly articulate. His mental weaknefs funk
him into fuch a ftate of torpitude, that he
muft have perifhed for food, had he not
been fed with all the care and attention that
is requifite for a baby.   He often flavered
from his mouth, ftood like a ftatue with
his eyes immoveably fixed on the ground,
and was not eafily to be removed from
that pofition.   His extremities were livid
and cold in the heat of fummer; his eyes
prominent, and appeared as if covered
with varnifh; the pupils were contracted, the cheeks fallen, and the nofe, particularly at the point, of a livid red, and
covered with carbuncles.   As the conftitution had been fo much impaired by
the frequent ufe of mercury, which had
caufed

caufed a confiderable diffolution of the
blood; and his nerves, naturally weak,
been reduced to extreme debility; I
put him under a courfe of mild alterative medicines, prefcribed a nutritious regimen, and enjoined the ftricteft
obfervation to cleanlinefs. After perfevering in this manner for fome months, by
repeated interrogation, I was now and
then able to obtain a fingle word from him
by way of anfwer. For the humour in
his face, a feton was made between the
fhoulders in the direction of the fpine,
which afforded a copious difcharge, and
was kept open for a confiderable time,
but to very little purpofe, as he continued
nearly in the fame ftate, except partially
recovering the ufe of his legs, for he could
but juft fet one foot before the other, and
creep a few paces with difficulty when at
the beft. He would fometimes take his
food without any affiftance; and although
he afterwards recovered fome fhare of
recollection, he was obliged to hefitate a
confiderable time before he could make
a pertinent reply to any one queftion that
was propofed to him. Thus from being a
fenfible

fenfible promifing young man, with the advantage of a liberal education, poffeffing a moft lively imagination with the moft acute fenfibility, from injudicious treatment at the commencement of his diforder, he became a melancholy fpectacle of fcarcely half animated exiftence; nor was he ever after capable of fulfilling the ordinary duties of life, or of undergoing the common familiar forms of focial intercourfe. Such are the pernicious effects of mercury, incautioufly adminiftered, to perfons of a weak and tender habit! and innumerable are the ferious mifchiefs occurring from taking cold, when under the influence of this powerful medicine.

CASE XLVIII.

A YOUNG gentleman, of a thin and delicate habit of body, from a fudden fright in his fifteenth year, was fuddenly feized with a coldnefs, quick and difficult refpiration, univerfal tremor, a diarrhœa, incontinence

of

of urine, and a contraction of his features; and although the caufe of his fear
was foon after removed, yet it had made
fuch a violent impreffion on his mind, as
to occafion a privation of his intellectual
powers.   He could not be brought to
himfelf, but laboured under extreme anxiety, fighed, and fhed tears; his hearing
was depraved; and he reeled about,
with his hand to his head, as if inebri-
ated.   Febrile fymptoms coming on, he
was put to bed, but neither perfpired
nor paffed any water, during two days
and nights.   Notwithftanding every medical affiftance was adminiftered, he never
afterwards recovered his fenfes; his
mind not poffeffing fufficient energy to
free itfelf from the exceffive agitation it
had experienced, although it is now a
confiderable time fince the accident; and
his memory and imagination are in that
ftate of diforganization and debility, as to
preclude all hopes of his recovery.

I have had the care and management of
this young man more than eight years,
who ftill in his afpect retains an expreffion
of that terror which the object firft excited;
and

and all the affiſtance I have been able to render him, has been from the repeated exhibition of emetics, to remove the prodigious quantity of phlegm with which he is apt to abound ; laxatives; though of the moſt gentle kind, having been found to weaken him beyond meaſure. And in the general treatment of mania, it muſt be allowed by thoſe who have had but a moderate ſhare of experience, that emetics are in general capable of affording more effential ſervice than cathartic remedies, and that the patient is generally much leſs debilitated by the former, than by the operation of the latter.

CASE XLIX.

A SUPPRESSION of the menſtrual flux, either from mental affeĉtions, viſcid adheſion in the blood, defeĉt of quantity, or from ſome accidental cauſe, is always attended with injury to the conſtitution, ſo far as even to induce inſanity, as will appear in the two ſubſequent caſes.

P. T.

P. T. a young lady of delicate conftitution, taking cold at a particular period in her eighteenth year, by imprudently fitting too long in her damp
cloaths, after having been accidentally wet
through in a fhower of rain, on the evening of the fame day was attacked with a
rigor, reftleffnefs, laffitude, and pain in
the loins, that was foon after fucceeded
by great heat, a frequent and full pulfe,
pain in the region of the womb, fwelling
and tenfion of the belly and ftomach, an
inclination to vomit, dry fkin, rednefs and
inflammation of the eyes, pains in the legs,
with great anxiety and depreffion of fpirits. The practitioner who was confulted
on this occafion, ordered a vomit, and on
the fucceeding morning took away ten
ounces of blood. An opiate was prefcribed
at bed-time, and at intervals an emulfion of
almonds, with the addition of nitre and
gum arabic. The fymptoms appeared in
fome degree mitigated; but on the third
day from the firft attack, great heat, thirft,
reftleffnefs, fpafms, and delirium occurred.
Farther medical affiftance became necef-

fary,

fary, by which means the acute continual fever was tranflated to a favourable crifis on the thirteenth day ; but the patient ftill complained of pain and weight in the head, with irrefolution, lofs of memory and recollection, deafnefs and dimnefs of fight; the functions of the mind were obvioufly impaired ; and as fhe recovered her bodily ftrength, fhe was frequently impelled to the commiffion of many ridiculous and abfurd actions. She grew impatient of controul, was bold, refolute, and loft to fhame ; her eyes were fuffufed with blood, on every flight and trifling occafion, fhe would fly into paffions contrary to her nature, and often fhed involuntary tears, fhe alternately laughed and fung, was fly and artful in her actions, and profane and lafcivious in her expreffions. Her appetite was exceedingly indifferent, and her digeftion remarkably difficult ; fhe was much emaciated, and œdematous fwellings affected her feet and ankles. Emmenagogues of different kinds had for fome months been adminiftered to reftore the menftrual evacuation ; to facilitate which purpofe,

purpofe, electricity had alfo been advifed, but to no effect; and at the latter end of November 1788, fhe was wholly confign- ed to my care. The pulfe was foft, flow, and weak; the circulation languid; her countenance white and bloated; and fhe was fubject to fpafms and tremors. I prefcribed a gentle antimonial emetic, that operated fo well as to bring from off the ftomach a quantity of phlegm and chocolate-coloured bile; the warm pedilu- vium was ufed every night, and a feton paffed between the fhoulders in the direc- tion of the fpine; the camphorated ace- tated mixture was prefcribed every morn- ing an hour before dinner, and at five o'clock in the afternoon, befides which fhe took every night and morning a bolus of the following form:

R Conferv. Rorifmarin.   3fs.
    Limiatur Chalyb.   gr. x.
    Pulv. Myrrh. Comp.   gr. xv.
    Pulv. Aromat.   gr. ij.
    Syr. e Cort. Aurant. q. f. f. bolus fuperbi-
bend. bol. fing. Cyathum Infuf. Rad Raphan. Ruftican.

This

This prefcription fhe continued to take from the 23d of November 1788, to the latter end of February 1789, an emetic being prefcribed at the interval of every nine or ten days at furtheft, and occafionally an omiffion of the bolus at night, on account of the turbulent and outrageous manner in which fhe behaved in the evening, that caufed the impracticability of its adminiftration. The firft re-appearance of the menfes was on the 27th of April, foon after which her health and ftrength vifibly recovered, and her reafon began to re-illumine; fhe became lefs violent and mifchievous, and was more eafily managed; her diforder evidently continued to leffen, and upon the fourth reflux of the menftrual difcharge that occurred regularly at the proper periods, fhe was fo much recovered as to be rendered fociable, and was in confequence admitted to join the family at meals, and at other times; where fhe conducted herfelf with propriety and decorum for upwards of nine years. Except a flight opthalmia, caufed from

obftructed

obftructed perfpiration, by getting wet in
in the feet, that was relieved in a few
days by bleeding and antiphlogiftic medicines, fhe had no fort of complaint till fhe
returned to her friends and relations in
Norfolk, where fhe has ever fince continued in perfect health, without experiencing the leaft fymptom of her former
mania.

CASE L.

A WOMAN, aged thirty, of a ftrong
conftitution, a choleric habit of body, and
violently paffionate difpofition, from a
fuppreffion of the menfes occafioned by a
fudden fit of anger, in the year 1780,
became infane. She was extremely outrageous, and fo powerful as to overcome
almoft every perfon with whom fhe had
any contention. She expreffed the moft
bitter abhorrence to thofe perfons with
whom fhe had lived many years in habits
of the moft friendly intimacy. But the
ftrong

ftrong and rooted impreffion that was
fixed in her mind, which was the original caufe of her complaint, evidently
appeared at all times to be predominant in her imagination; and for
three years fucceffively fhe was not able
to fubdue this propenfity; nor did fhe
once menftruate in all that time, although fhe had been unremittingly regular
in that refpect during feveral years before.   When fhe was fent to me, fhe had
the hæmorrhoids to a very violent degree;
and fhe had been fo much permitted to
have her own way, that nothing was fo
great a punifhment to her as reftriction.
The confequence of which was, that fhe
had been fuffered to indulge in thofe kinds
of food that were moft prejudicial to
her diforder; and would not fuffer herfelf
to be kept decently clean, or be prevailed
on to take fuch medicines as were beft
calculated to diminifh her affliction.   Her
converfation was confined to one object.
She was coftive, and had a dry cough; her
countenance was florid; and fhe was continually loud, loquacious, or impertinently
communicative.   The pulfe was hard and
ftrong;

ftrong ; fhe was noify and reftlefs of
nights; and her fkin was harfh and dry.
To deplete the veffels, and attenuate the
humours, I ordered ten ounces of blood
to be taken from the arm, that, when
cold, was covered with a yellow encrufted
fize ; lenient purgatives were occafionally
adminiftered ; a feton was paffed between the fhoulders in the direction of
the fpine. After a fortnight I ordered
the bleeding to be repeated ; with a
mode of treatment, and regimen, exact-
ly the reverfe of what fhe had been
accuftomed to. The warm pediluvium
was ufed every night, and fhe went
through a courfe of mild mercurial alteratives, that after continuing nearly nine
weeks, caufed the bodily fymptoms' to
vanifh, and evident figns of fanity to appear. During a period of twelve months
fhe menftruated freely and regularly
without interruption; fhe was permitted
to return to her former habitation; and
by ftrictly adhering to the medical advice
that was given her, upon leaving my
houfe, and abiding by the rules prefcribed

for

for the government of her paſſions, ſhe
has ſince continued well without experiencing any kind of relapſe.

CASE LI.

A GENTLEMAN, about fifty, who
for more than nine years had been ſubject to hypochondriacal inſanity, was
through its influence reduced to a variety of painful and diſagreeable ſenſations,
almoſt without intermiſſion, the laſt four
years of which he had been under my
care. In July 1785, he was ſuddenly
ſeized with an acute pain in the head,
back, and loins, a wearineſs in his limbs,
and general laſſitude pervaded his whole
frame; ſhivering and coldneſs in the extremities; ſtretching, yawning, ſickneſs
with vomiting and heat, thirſt, and fever,
ſucceeded. His ſkin became moiſt, a
profuſe ſweat, and a confirmed intermittent was the conſequence. After eleven
ſucceſſive paroxyſms, that had returned
every

every third day, by the affiftance of emetics and bark, the diforder was entirely
fubdued, and he was effectually cured of
his fever and infanity at the fame time,
and has ever fince remained entirely free
from both.   Two fimilar inftances have
fince occurred in my practice.

In Dr. Monro's remarks on Dr. Battie's Treatife on Madnefs, he has mentioned three cafes of intermittent fever occurring to fome perfons who had
been mad for many years ; two of which
he affirms to have feen himfelf, where the
cure of one proved alfo the cure of the
other.

CASE LII.

A. M. a gentleman of fortune, habitually intemperate in his way of living, fubject to regular fits of the gout, and to an
hereditary afthma of the humoral kind,
having had no return of arthritic affection
for nearly two years, became fuddenly

P   low-

low-fpirited, with great diftrefs and anxiety of mind; every trifling occurrence
was confidered by him as an objeét of intenfe trouble and inquietude, he was dif-
gufted with almoft every thing and every
body, and entirely rejeéted thofe enjoy-
ments and relaxations of life that had before given him the greateft pleafure and
fatisfaétion; and in a fhort time, his mind
was funk into the loweft abyfs of melancholy and dejeétion.

It is extraordinary, that from the very
commencement of mental derangement,
he was totally exempt from the afthmatic
complaint, and continued fo from the beginning of February 1785 till the latter
end of November following, when he
complained of drowfinefs, languor, and
dullnefs, attended with rigors and ficknefs; and foon after was attacked with
pains in his feet, ankles, and the calves of
his legs; when in a few hours he became as
clear in his imagination and fenfes as ever
he had been in his life, and continued fo
throughout the whole gouty period of almoft nine weeks; during which interval the
afthmatic

afthmatic diforder, as he became infane, receded, as it had done before. He now expreffed the moft violent refentment againft his neareft relations, was mifchievous in his defigns againft himfelf, and would certainly have committed fuicide had he not been carefully prevented. Thus he continued under the influence of the moft defperate infanity, until the latter end of the following April, when he was feized with a fhivering, and flight fever, that was fucceeded by a regular fit of the gout, exempt from the afthmatic complaint, which was attended with the fame intellectual clearnefs and perfpicuity as before, and again recurred upon the declenfion of the gouty paroxyfm, which again left him a prey to the ravages of mental derangement, and afthmatic affections.

In this ftate he was removed from my care; and the laft information I heard concerning him was that he had experienced no return of the gout during a period of twelve months, that his lungs were in a very weak ftate, attended with a wafting of every part of his body, in-

dicative

dicative of a general decay; and that foon
after he was attacked with a gouty dyfen-
tery, which terminated in an abfcefs of the
bowels, and occafioned his death.

C A S E   LIII.

G. H. a man in the thirty-eighth year of
his age, by trade a brafs-wire-drawer, thin,
bilious, of low ftature, and fallow complexion, was at intervals afflicted with
violent pains in his bowels, particularly
about the navel, attended with confiderable diftenfion of the abdomen, and often
with contractions of the mufcles of the
belly. The caufe of his complaint being
at its commencement attributed to wind,
he took feveral carminative medicines,
but feldom with any other effect than of
increafing his uneafinefs. Thefe pains,
after continuing about an hour, gradually
decreafed, until they entirely fubfided.
He was attacked with this paroxyfm every
day, generally about the fame hour, that
was ufually preceded by a violent itching
of

of the nofe, a tingling in the ears, and a
fenfation of heat and tenfion in the right
hypochondrium. During the attack he
complained of thirft, was giddy, and fometimes very fick at his ftomach. He had
confulted an eminent phyfician in town,
who attributed the complaint partly to
the nature of the bufinefs which he was
obliged to follow, and partly to an hypochondriacal affection.

From what I could learn, the nature of
his prefcription was the pil. galbani
comp. caftor and opium, preceded by an
emetic. From thefe medicines he derived
no fervice, and foon after his ideas were
difcovered to be vague, confufed, and unconnected, paffing in rapid fucceffion, without regularity or order. A confirmed hypochondriac melancholy afterwards occurred, when in a moft diftrefsful tone of voice
he would often affure the by-ftanders
that he was made of glafs, and was
fearful of moving leaft he fhould break
to pieces. He continued in this ftate
during fome weeks, without either the
affiftance of medicine, a regimen fuitable

to

to his cafe, or that kind of management
which was apparently neceffary for his
relief. On the 17th of May 1785, I was
confulted, and found that he enjoyed
but little fleep of a night; the faculties
of his mind were much impaired; his memory almoft annihilated; he had frequent
palpitations of the heart, with anxiety,
fighing, indigeftion, and hypochondriacal
languor; was fubject to congeftions of
vifcid matter in the ftomach; had chilly
fweats, flatulencies, and eructations; was
pale, emaciated, weak, and inclined to be
coftive. There appeared an uncommon
vacancy in his looks, with a tremulous
vibration of the eye-lids; he obftinately
perfevered in the idea that he was made of
glafs, and upon the leaft motion dreaded
that he fhould be fhivered to pieces. This
opinion made him almoft motionlefs, and
he appeared like one in the catalepfy; he
never moved either hand or foot, without
the greateft caution and deliberation; his
voice was fmall, timid, and indiftinct; his
pofition in general fupine, with his hands
and legs extended; the pulfe was flender

and

and intermitted every third or fourth
ftroke; his refpiration difficult; the urine
variable, fometimes turbid and milky, and
at others was obferved to have fine threads
in it refembling bits of fpider's webs, and
at others depofiting a light fediment; his
ftools were fometimes frequent, bilious,
loofe, and fœtid, at others coftive, and of
the colour of clay. There was a continual tumour and tenfion of the abdomen,
with a rumbling of the inteftines. His
eyes were hollow, the pupils diftended and
the eye-lids puffed and livid; his breath
was unufually fœtid, ftrong, and offenfive;
from which I was induced to think that
worms, from their irritation of the inteftines, might have produced the debility
in the firft paffages, and have been the
primary caufe of his diforder. Upon the
ftrifteft inquiry I could not find that
the patient had ever been fufpefted to
have been afflifted with worms, or had
ever voided any. But fully poffeffed of
this opinion, from having feen children
fubjefted to fpafms and delirium from
the irritation occafioned in the ftomach
and

and inteftines by thefe reptiles, I directed
the following ointment to be applied warm
to the umbilical region :

> ℞ Fellis Bovi,
>   Aloes aa ℈j.
>   Ungt. Alb. Camph. ℈ij. M. f. Ungt.

and alfo ordered a decoction of quick-
filver in water, an ounce to a pint, to be
given him for his common drink, and the
following draught to be taken every
morning:

> ℞ Ol. Ricini.
>   Aq. Fontan. aa. ℈ij.
>   Tinct. Fœtid. ℈fs. M. f. Hauft.
> omni mane jejun. Ventriculo exhibend.

In the evening of the fourth day from the
beginning of this courfe, he voided by ftool
two large round thick worms of the
teretes kind; and the next day a third
much larger, rounder, and longer than the
two former.   As it was now no longer a
doubt that the exciting caufe of his delirium was from vermicular affection, and his
ftrength would now admit of it, more powerful anthelmintics were prefcribed with an
                                    occafional

occafional dofe of calomel and jalap at proper intervals, till his health was entirely reftored, and his reafon fo far recovered as to enable him to exercife his bufinefs as ufual.

Although thefe medicines were not entirely difcontinued for fome confiderable time, I did not hear of his voiding any other worms; therefore had the greateft reafon to conclude, that the vermicular fac was totally deftroyed by their anthelminthic power, efpecially fo as he has ever fince continued free from any mental complaint whatever.

CASE LIV.

IN the latter end of the year 1784, I was fent for to a gentleman of great eminence in the commercial line. He was about forty years of age, of a fcorbutic habit of body, with predifpofition to infanity. I was informed by the gentleman who

attended

attended him, that in the autumn of the
fame year, when the fcarlet fever and fore
throat proved epidemic in the town where
he lived, he was feized with ficknefs at the
ftomach, laffitude, and fhivering; complained of a violent head-ach, heat, pain,
and tenfion in the throat; his fkin became harfh and hot; the pulfe was quick,
ftrong, and hard, with preternatural heat,
and the functions of the brain were much difturbed; his deglutition became painful and
exceffively difficult; the tonfils, and uvula
appeared inflamed and furrounded with
white floughs and ulcerations; the mouth
and fauces were covered with mucus, and
there was a confiderable tumefaction in
the throat; the fcarlet efflorefcence appeared on the third day after the attack,
tinged the fkin of a dufky red colour, and
was diffufed over the whole body, with
œdematous fwellings of the hands and
feet. The warm pediluvium was ufed,
and the emetic tartar adminiftered, that
operated by ftool and vomit; the fauces
were cleanfed by warm detergent gargles;
and by a fubfequent courfe of tonic medicines

cines with proper laxatives, the patient recovered.   But his conduct and behaviour
were foon afterwards obferved to be very
diffimilar to what they were antecedent to
his illnefs.   His ideas were vague, wild,
and incoherent; his imagination depraved
and perverted ; and his judgment apparently under the influence of difeafed perceptions.

In this firft ftage of infanity, a blifter
was applied between the fhoulders, antimonial emetics were repeatedly adminiftered,
the warm bath was ufed, and many
other means adopted to very little, if
any, effect.   He became the victim of
various oppofite paffions ; was loft in
fpeculation, and fcarcely ever appeared to know or attend to any external object.   He flept little, and was fo
very turbulent and mifchievous, that it
became neceffary for a perfon continually
to watch his actions.

At this period of the diforder I firft
faw him.   His breath was hot and offenfive ; he had almoft a continual rumbling
of his bowels ; a catarrh, with frequent
fneezings,

ſneezings, and a dry cough from habitual indigeſtion. He was ridiculouſly timid, or violently bold and loquacious. The urine either pale and in ſmall quantities, or turbid and high-coloured. He was obſtinately coſtive, deaf, and inattentive. There was either a ſtupid vacancy in his manner and appearance, or an unnatural briſkneſs and protuberance of the eyes; he frequently uttered with the greateſt volubility ſome unconnected and unintelligible jargon; was ſubject to violent eructations, often foamed at the mouth, and ſpat indiſcriminately on all ſides of him, on any perſon or thing that ſtood in his way. The pulſe was hard, ſtrong, and quick; but his reſpiration tolerably free and eaſy. I directed twelve ounces of blood to be taken from his arm, that was grumous, black, and thick, with ſalt ſerum and a greeniſh mucus on the ſurface; a ſeton was alſo paſſed between the ſhoulders in the direction of the ſpine; and the following preſcription left with his apothecary:

℞ Antim.

℞ Antim. Tart. gr. iv.

Sacch. Alb. ℥ij. M. et f. Pulvis cujus fu_
mat grana feptim. mane & vefpere capiat Cyath. men-
fur. larg. Mift. Camphorat. acetat. intermediis fpatiis
5ta vel 6ta quaq. hora et Decoɛti Furfuris bibat ad
libitum.

The regimen was ordered to be cooling
and laxative, and chiefly to confift of vegetables. Finding him confiderably better in every refpeɛt, the next vifit I paid
him I advifed the continuance of the
medicines and regimen. The feton difcharged exceedingly well, and was attended with good effeɛt. By degrees he became tolerably rational at the end of fix
weeks, when he was fuddenly attacked
with the gout in his hands, which was carried off for the prefent by fuitable remedies and regimen; but his mind was in
too feeble a ftate to admit of his conduɛt-
ing his affairs with his ufual order and
propriety; and which it is much to be
feared he will never again be able to ac-
complifh. Since its firft vifit the gout has
regularly returned every fpring and fall, at
which times his intelleɛts are cleareft, and
he is tolerably rational and focial, but at
other

other times fly, gloomy, and fufpicious, and averfe to all kinds of company and converfation.

It is remarkable, that very few maniacs who have been fubject to periodical returns of rheumatifm or gout, fuffer much from either of thofe diforders afterwards; or that whenever fuch paroxyfms do return, their reafon feldom becomes ameliorated beyond the exiftence of the fit, and fometimes not even then.

CASE LV.

IN the cafe of this patient it may be obferved that there was an hereditary difpofition to madnefs.   He was of an extenuated form, and delicate habit of body. The tone of the vafcular fyftem had been enfeebled by an indolent and fedentary life.   For fome time paft he had been afflicted with the piles, attended with flatulencies, indigeftion, obtufe pains in the right hypochondrium under the fhort ribs;

ribs; anxiety, depraved appetite, coſtive-
neſs, with a cough and expectoration which
was ſometimes tinged with blood; a ſwelled
face, with deafneſs and a ſenſe of weight in
the head and dimneſs of ſight, attended
with ſymptoms of inſanity, which for a
time were not ſo violent, but that he
knew and could diſtinguiſh ſurrounding
objects.   At length he became entirely
inſane; and I never remember to have
heard a maniac queſtion and anſwer with
ſuch an animated velocity.   This was the
more extraordinary, as I was well informed
by thoſe who had long been acquainted
with him, that his natural intellectual
powers were below the ſtandard of medio-
crity, and rather feeble and contracted
than otherwiſe; but now what Shakeſpear
obſerves in Hamlet, was extremely appo-
ſite to the ſituation of this maniac:

" How pregnant his replies!
" A happineſs that madneſs often hits on,
" The which fancy and reaſon would not be
" So proſperouſly delivered of."

As the pulſe ſufficiently indicated the neceſſity of the operation, eight ounces of
blood

blood were taken from the arm, the complexion of which afforded but little information; but rather indicated inflammation than otherwife, after giving fome directions for the regulation of his diet, to remove the congeftion of vifcid matter in the ftomach, with which it had long been too replete, an emetic was adminiftered, and afterwards an emulfion of almonds, nitre, gum arabic, manna, and foluble tartar; a feton was alfo made between the fhoulders in the direction of the fpine, and the warm pediluvium conftantly ufed at bed-time. He took the camphorated acetated mixture three times a day, and had a blifter applied to the right hypochondrium. Five days after the firft operation, the fame quantity of blood was taken from him as before, and in a few days he recovered much of his natural appearance, and was much lefs volatile and fluent in his expreffions and replies. The coftivenefs and hæmorrhoids were removed, and his appetite, that was never very confiderable, increafed. The cough never left him, and

in

in fix weeks he recovered his hearing and fight; and by the ufe of tonics, fea-air, bathing, and proper exercife, the fun&ions of his mind were reftored to their priftine ftate, and he remained confiderably better for feveral months; when getting cold, and being attacked with an eryfipetalous humour in his head and face, that was too haftily repelled by a topical application, recommended by an ignorant Dabbler in Phyfic, his maniacal fymptoms returned. In this ftate he continued a much longer time than before; and although a lucid interval of confiderable length fucceeded, yet his rational faculties had fuftained too much injury to render him capable of fulfilling the ordinary duties of life, of properly condu&ing himfelf in focial intercourfe, or of being trufted with the difpofal of his own perfon and fortune.

Q   C A S E

CASE LVI.

IT were to difregard the teftimony of truth, to deny that a continual courfe of intoxication, not only induces, but haftens the approach of infanity. From the many cafes of madnefs I have known to be produced by inebriation, I have felected the following, as a ufeful memento to thofe who perfevere in this deftructive and pernicious practice, fo very fubverfive and derogatory to the dignity of the human character.

In the month of October 1784, I was defired to attend a gentleman whofe nervous fyftem had been much injured, and whofe memory was almoft annihilated by exceffive drinking. He was a man of natural ftrong and lively paffions; in the early part of his life he had lived temperately and abftemioufly, and was much efteemed by his friends and acquaintance for his honour, induftry, and integrity; but from an habitual courfe of drinking he had neglected the focial virtues, and become infane. By proper

treatment

treatment he recovered, after having remained in this truly melancholic situation
for three weeks; but soon after returning
to his former habit of reiterated intoxication, a general plenitude and grossness of
habit ensued, and his health apparently began to decline. A train of hypochondriacal affections succeeded; his nights were
restless, his sleep perturbed. He complained of habitual languor and dejection of
spirits; his melancholic state of mind was
always obvious when not exhilarated with
liquor; and more than once, in a state of
despondency, he had endeavoured to commit suicide, which he certainly would have
accomplished, had he not been fortunately
prevented. In his fits he was violent, outrageous, insolent, and abusive; and in this
state, without obtaining any sleep, or even
being undressed, he continued sixteen days
and nights. At the desire of his relations,
and by my advice, he was put under such
restrictions as were absolutely necessary as
the preliminary to a regimen the very re-
verse of that to which he had too long been
accustomed. The tone of his whole frame

was

was fhattered and debilitated ; his features were bloated; his belly hard and tenfe; his breath hot and offenfive; his whole fyftem was convulfed ; he was violently delirious, and all over in a tremor. His eyes were dif-torted and inflamed; he had a hiccough, with lofs of voice and ftupidity, and a yellow caft over the whole furface of his fkin. His tongue was tremulous and black, and his ftools were paffed involuntarily. In this hopelefs ftate it was in vain to expect relief, either from medicine or management, and he fell a martyr to his intemperance on the fourth day after I vifited him.

CASE LVII.

As the preceding cafe exhibits the moft ftriking inftance of the fatal effects which proceed from that pernicious habit, exceffive drinking, the following is inferted as an encouragement to the intemperate to defift from this vicious courfe before the foundation of the conftitution is

fo

so entirely sapped of its natural vigour as to produce the most certain and inevitable destruction. Innumerable are the evils that are in the train of this vice.

It was about four years ago that I was applied to concerning a gentleman about five-and-forty years of age, naturally of an acute and painful sensation, and of a corpulent make, but relaxed fibres; who for two years past had habitually addicted himself to drinking spirituous liquors to excess; the consequences of which were indolence, debility, languor, palpitation at the heart, uneasy respiration, vertigo, and apepsia. He became unsteady and untoward in his conduct, hostile to advice, weak in judgment, defective in memory, and shewed evident signs of a disordered imagination. Want of appetite, nausea, and great weakness of the stomach ensued, with tremors, fear, apprehension, and distressful feelings. He complained of heat and pain in the right hypochondrium, loss of memory, a singing noise in his ears, and had an epileptic fit; on recovering from which a total want of sleep supervened, and the derange-

derangement of his mind was fuch as to require the greateft care and precaution of thofe about him to prevent his perpetrating any mifchief to himfelf and others.

When I firft faw him, he had obtained no fleep for feven nights fucceffively, and his bodily complaints were fo vifibly accompanied with that horror and defpair of countenance, as to remind me of an appropriate application from Spenfer:

> " Ever fitting on the ground,
> " Mufing full fadly in his fullen mind;
> " His grifly locks long grown and unbound,
> " Difordered hung almoft his fhoulders round
> " And hid his face————."

His countenance was florid; he was un-fteady in his walking; there was a vacant ftaring appearance in his eyes, that were much diftorted, and the pupils greatly enlarged; he had a quick full pulfe; his tongue was white and dry; the mufcles of his arms and legs were emaciated; his bowels were in an exceffive ftate of confti-pation, and apparently diftended with wind; he appeared at times much tor-mented with pain, which he expreffed by

bending

bending himfelf double, rigidly contracting the mufcles of his face, and biting his
under lip till it bled.   I prefcribed bleeding, and endeavoured to procure a free
paffage for the excrements by repeated
dofes of kali tartar.; and that failing, recourfe was had to a ftimulating clyfter,
which anfwered the intended purpofe for
the prefent, after which, by mild aperient
medicines and a fuitable diet, the bowels
were kept in a proper ftate of laxity; but
a dangerous diarrhœa coming on, in which
his ftools were frequent, thin, and fharp,
moft urgent in the night, notwithftanding
the maniacal fymptoms, I ventured upon
the ufe of opiates, with rad. rhei and requifite aftringents; after having cleanfed
the ftomach with a few grains of ipecacuanha, by which means, after a few days,
it was entirely removed.   But the fame
derangement of mind continued as at firft,
and influenced him alternately with vehement paffions, loud mirth, or deep dejection, grief, and fettled melancholy.   His
urine fometimes paffed involuntarily, but
his ftools never; he had frequent fpafmodic

dic pains in his arms, and a flight paraly-
fis in the left leg, that was in confequence
almoft deprived of its motion; it was
embrocated with the liniment faponis,
which proved highly efficacious. He had
frequently fo obftinate a retention of the
fœces, that his ftools were procured with
difficulty. A blifter was applied to the
leg, a feton paffed between the fhoulders
in the direction of the fpine, the warm
pediluvium applied conftantly at bed time,
and a bolus compofed of camphor, valerian, and muftard adminiftered twice a
day.

This courfe he had continued about
three weeks, when the good effects were
mánifeft, his leg was reftored to its ufe,
and his health nearly recovered. It being a proper feafon of the year for ufing
the waters, he went to Bath, accompanied
by a near relation; and in a few weeks
his bodily health was reftored, and no
trace of any infane fymptom remained.
Being now convinced how much he would
be expofed to a relapfe, by reverting to
the deftructive cuftom that had been the
caufe

caufe of his difordered mind, he became
unremittingly abftemious, and diligent in
the ftrict obfervance of temperance in
diet, and the proper regulation of his
paffions, the natural confequence of which
was uninterrupted health and undifeafed
idea.

CASE LVIII.

THE fubftance of this cafe was circum-
ftantially related to me by letter, dated
Minories, London, June 21ft, 1785, in
which it appears that the caufe and effect of this patient's infanity proceeded
from the fuppreffion of an old ulcer in
the leg, with which fhe had been afflicted
upwards of fix years, Through the
bilious quality of her blood, fhe was naturally of a phlegmatic, cold habit, and had
long been under the care of a judicious
furgeon, who enjoined a proper regimen,
and treated her according to the indication of her cafe.   Notwithftanding the
ulcer remained ftubborn and troublefome,
                                    and

and was accompanied with a large difcharge, nor could the endeavours of feveral gentlemen of the faculty caufe its ma-
lignancy to abate. She had never been
ftrictly regular in her menftrual periods,
and having heard of an empirical pre-
tender to medicine, who fhe had been informed had accomplifhed many wonderful
cures in fimilar cafes, and defpairing of
otherwife experiencing relief, fhe very
readily determined to abide by his advice.
In about fix weeks afterwards, by his
extraordinary fkill and knowledge, the
difcharge from the ulcer was wholly fuppreffed, and it entirely healed. This apparent fuccefs gained the practitioner no
inconfiderable degree of credit, as having
wrought an unprecedented and almoft
miraculous cure. But his newly-acquired
fame was but of fhort duration; for
three weeks had fcarcely elapfed, before fhe was attacked with a variety of
hyfterical fymptoms, and fuch other complaints as conclufively degenerated into a
confirmed mania, too generally to be
dreaded as the confequence of haftily fup-
preffing by art thofe morbid difcharges
which

which having become habitual, relieve the conftitution, and enfure that fhare of health which is only the effect of nature's efforts to free herfelf from that which is obnoxious to the conftitution; and where no other drain has been fubftituted in the room of that which has been fuppreffed, the effects of repletion will foon become confpicuous in a variety of morbid appearances. It was only in this diforder fhe laboured with extreme anxiety, fear, and diftrefs of mind; talked incoherently, raved, was furious, and had little or no fleep. She was coftive, the abdomen was tenfe, and her breath extremely offenfive. She had frequently fpafmodic contractions of the joints, and appeared much more deaf than before fhe was attacked with thefe maniacal fymptoms. She had an eruption of the eryfipetalous kind in her face, the pupils of her eyes were much enlarged, and her eye-lids fwelled and inflamed. She was fubject to acid eructations, and often expectorated a thick purulent matter. Her eyes were in conftant motion;

fhe

fhe had often a loud palpitation of the heart; was conftantly changing her pofition; the pulfe was quick, ftrong, and hard, with confiderable preternatural heat. Her refpiration was difficult, her fkin harfh, fqualid, and dry. Her diet had been exceedingly improper for a perfon in her fituation; therefore an alteration of it was immediately recommended, to attenuate the nature of the fluids, and fhe loft twelve ounces of blood from the arm. A feton was paffed between the fhoulders in the direction of the fpine, and an iffue was opened below the knee in the leg that had been ulcerated; an emetic was adminiftered on the third day after I faw her, which brought away a great quantity of bile and phlegm; on the fucceeding day fix drachms of foluble tartar were adminiftered, which was occafionally repeated, and by way of alterative the following pill:

R Mercur. calcinat. ℈fs.

Ocul. Cauci. ppt.

Conferv. Rofar. aa. ℈j. M. f. Pil. xx.

Quorum fumat ij omni Nocte H. S. fuperbibend. Cyathum Mift Camph. acetata et aquæ puræ p. æ. mift.

In

In this courfe fhe had continued with very little alteration for nearly five weeks, when the catamenia appeared, although not in great quantity, the maniacal fymptoms abated, in lefs than three weeks after which the difcharge returned again to its former extent, and continued its regularity for fome months. She became fo well as to be trufted by herfelf, could read, write, and converfe as rationally as ever; and by the occafional affiftance of a little medicine, has continued perfectly well ever fince. The feton has been dried up fome time, but the iffue in her leg continues open, and difcharges very well.

CASE LIX.

COMMUNICATED in a letter from a lady.

" Sir,

" THE following cafe is of a perfon whofe whole fupport is on her own induftry; and I fhould be much obliged to
you

you for your opinion on it, and a prefcription for her to follow. She is a very
worthy woman in her ftation, I fhould be
happy to relieve her. She was pretty
nearly in the fame way five-and-twenty
years ago, and has had no return fince.
Mrs. S. J. feventy-four years of age, was
attacked in March laft, with an irregular
fever, flight pain in the cheft under the fternum, flatulency in the ftomach and bowels, much depreffion of fpirit, fome anxiety, fome degree of thirft, lies with her
eyes fhut, talks abfurdly, tumbles and
toffes about with a great inclination to
fleep without being able to obtain it. Various febrifuge and neurotic medicines
were for fome time given, but without
effect; a blifter was applied to the head,
and a vomit was intended, but objected to
on account of her great deformity of body.
The faline mixture, fp. mindereri pulv.
contray. c. caftor crocus pil. fœtid. and
cortex peruv. were given as the variation
of the fymptoms feemed to indicate, but
the diforder increafed, and for ten or
twelve weeks fhe had funk into a religious
defpondency,

defpondency, accompanied either with unremitting fervours of zeal and devotion,
or incredible expectations of divine manifeftations, much emotion and ardour on
the groundlefs fear and apprehenfion that
fhe had incurred the refentment of the
Deity, and fhall hereafter undergo the
punifhment of the moft hardened and atro-
cious finner, although there has been no
part of her life open to blame, or in the
leaft governed by irregular gratification, but on the contrary, pure and im-
maculate in thought, word, and deed.
From thefe diftreffing ideas nothing can
rouze or divert her mind, although fhe
converfes rationally, but reluctantly, on
any other fubject. Her appetite is good,
her pulfe in general too quick, without
fulnefs. The tongue in moft part moift ;
the body inclined to coftivenefs ; the urine
natural, both in colour and quantity, but
feldom depofiting any fediment ; fhe has
fometimes perfpired pretty freely in the
night, but generally found herfelf more
relaxed the enfuing day. No medicines
have been given her for five or fix weeks,
except

except through neceffity, fomething laxative.

I am, &c."

Portman-Square,
June 30th, 1786.

THE ANSWER.

" Madam,

" AT her time of life I fear but little
can be done to affift the patient, whofe
cafe you have fo obligingly fubmitted to
my infpection and confideration. If fhe
could be converfed with on any regular
plan, her miftaken notions of religion
might probably be corrected; but in the
religious melancholy I have repeatedly
found that argument has had but little
weight, for it feems to be the nature of
the diforder to involve the mind in the
moft miferable and inextricable myfteries.
The patients thus influenced, refift or
evade every argument which the moft fenfible perfon can adduce from the moft
rational ground, to undeceive their blind-
ed judgment and deluded mind.   Perhaps
it

it were beſt to perſuade her that the effects
of her mind entirely originate from bodily
complaint.   It is pretty generally obſerved, that perſons who labour under fanatical inſanity, uſually die of a ſlow fever.
Perhaps ſhe is not altogether inclined to
company, although ſhe may be to buſineſs
or amuſement.   The mind, if poſſible,
ſhould be diverted, and kept in a calm
unruffled ſtate; and all converſation on
her favourite topic be carefully avoided.
Electricity might be uſeful to her : there
can be no hurt in trying it.   Friction of
the legs, arms, and trunk of the body, and
even of the belly, with a fleſh-bruſh, is ad-
viſeable, as thereby perſpiration might be
encouraged, and the circulation quickened.
She ſhould riſe early, and uſe as much exerciſe as the ſtrength and formation of her
body will admit.   I would adviſe ſix
grains of camphor and four of nitre, with
three grains of the powder of ſquills, made
into a bolus, with conſerve of roſemary, to
be taken every morning, noon, and night;
and with a view to relieve her typho-

R   mania,

mania, fhe may take a cupful of camphorated mixture, and repeat it as often
in the night as occafion may require. The
ol. ricini I would advife as a proper laxative: the dofes to be adminiftered by thofe
who are acquainted with her ftrength and
habit. Indeed it appears highly neceffary
that her body fhould be kept in a moderate cool and open ftate. Reclining her
head over the fteams of hot vinegar, in
which a quantity of myrrh, camphor, and
rofemary flowers have been infufed, may
be very ferviceable, and may be repeated
at thofe times when the fervour or horror
is moft prevalent. The deformity of her
fhape may probably afford a reafonable
objection to an emetic, or it would certainly have been right to have given one.
When you may think proper to write to
me again, the favour will be honourably
efteemed by,

Madam, &c."

In a few weeks after I had fent the
above advice, I had the fatisfaction to
hear

hear that my directions had been put into practice, and that the patient had found confiderable relief.

———————

CASE LX.

A. G. the mafter of a coafting veffel, about thirty-nine years of age, of a warm paffionate difpofition, an atrabilious conftitution, which had fuffered from the too liberal ufe of fpirituous liquors; and of a frame of mind eafily fufceptible of terror; being at fea a few leagues from fhore, was fuddenly terrified by a luminous appearance in the air, refembling, as he believed, a woman of gigantic ftature, arrayed in white and fplendid garments, of a threatening afpect, and moft tremendous countenance: this made fo deep an impreffion on his mind, as almoft inftantly to bereave him of his fenfes; and it was with great difficulty that he was fecured and brought on fhore, without committing fome act of felfviolence, which in his fits of defperation he

seemed

feemed obftinately determined on ; and had he not been fortunately prevented, would have terminated his exiftence by his own hand. He was a ftrong, powerful, mufcular man, and when brought to my houfe, it required three ftout perfons to manage him, notwithftanding he was at the fame time fecured in a ftrait-waiftcoat. Indeed he had attained the moft outrageous degree of raving madnefs. His refpiration was hard and difficult ; he had got no fleep from the time he received the fhock, which was about a week ; he frequently fhivered, as if with cold, and was fometimes drawn with univerfal convulfions ; had a moft extraordinary ferocity in his eyes, the tunica albuginea of which was ftreaked with red ; in the corners was a fordid rheum, and the pupils were much diftended ; his countenance was bloated, and of a crimfon hue ; he had a quick and full pulfe ; his tongue white and tremulous ; he foamed at the mouth ; and the teeth and lips were covered with a thick fordes, with rather a greafy appearance of the whole face ;

the

the features of which Lavater himfelf
might have delineated, with all the combined traits of fear, horror, and defpair. At intervals he appeared more
calm and eafy, and would anfwer, although indiftinctly and confufedly, fuch
queftions as were propofed to him ; but
the mind could not relieve itfelf of the
violent preffure which it had fuftained, and
he often relapfed into fuch fits of rage and
defperation, as were really terrible ; and
poffeffed fuch an invincible propenfity to
fuicide, that it was with difficulty he was
prevented from beating out his brains
againft the wall, or upon the floor ; and
notwithftanding his hands and legs were
well fecured, and he was confined in a
cell, in one of thofe frantic paroxyfms
he actually beat his head againft the bed-
ftead fo violently, that it remained a doubt
with us for fome time whether he had
not fractured his fkull, or occafioned a
concuffion of the brain ; and it was a long
time before he recovered from the effects
of this violence, which bringing on an abfcefs, that extended from the vertex to

the

the inferior part of the occiput, and
terminated in a profufe fuppuration,
that put a period to his maniacal complaint, by clearing the habit of its obnoxious humours; and at the end of two
months, being thoroughly reftored to his
intellectual faculties, he returned to his
family, convinced of the prudence and
indeed the neceffity of a more temperate
courfe of life.   He ftill continues his ufual
avocations undifeafed either in body or
mind.

CASE LXI.

SIMILAR in fome refpects to the foregoing is the following inftance of mania
furibunda, in John Munn, an alehoufe-
keeper in the parifh of Maidftone.   He
had long drank to excefs, and contracted
an habitual ftate of intoxication.   In June,
1799, he was taken with a complaint in his
ftomach, and depraved appetite, with bilious vomiting; and the apothecary applied

to,

to, imagining the complaint to proceed entirely from hard drinking, fent him an emetic, with fome ftomachic medicines, which were for fome time thought of fervice to him; but towards the end of the month he was taken worfe, with fymptoms of hypochondriafis, great reftleffnefs, pain in his head, anxiety, impaired tafte, indigeftion, and flight maniacal delirium. A phyfician was now confulted, who prefcribed bleeding. The blood was rather fizy; he then prefcribed an aperient medicine, with a continuation of the camphorated nervous medicines he had before taken; notwithftanding the patient got worfe, had a peculiar afpect, with a wild defponding look, and frantic manner; but when fpoke to, anfwered every queftion rationally. The maniacal fymptoms were now obferved to be moft violent during the night, and particularly after fleep (whenever he got any). Dreadful apprehenfions and great agonies at thofe times afflicted him. Two or three men that ufually fat up with him, were with difficulty able to keep him in the room; he had made feveral attempts

at

at fuicide, and fo violently beat and bruifed one of his attendants, that his life was for fome time defpaired of.

On the 19th of Auguft he had broke from his confinement, and thrown himfelf into a deep pond of water, with intent to drown himfelf, which he would certainly have effected had he not been timely obferved and dragged out by the hair of his head. Almoft immediately after this circumftance he was brought to my houfe in a ftrait-waiftcoat, that he foon after found means to get off, and with the ftrings and arms of which he hung himfelf up by the neck; but being again timely difcovered, was cut down, and thus preferved a fecond time from immediate felf-deftruction, but was not reftored to life till after many fevere fymptoms of fuffocation; and there remained a deep indenture in his neck for fome weeks afterwards, occafioned by his fufpenfion. Soon after this the patient, who was an uncommonly mufcular fquare-fet man, and poffeffed of incredible ftrength, which was increafed by his diforder, be-

came

came more furious and ungovernable than
before, and it was with the greateſt difficulty that he was ſecured by ſix ſtout
men; and although made as ſecure as the
nature of the caſe would admit, he found
means to beat his elbows againſt the ſide
of the cell with ſuch determined violence as to occaſion the blood to ſtream
through his clothes, proteſting the moſt
dreadful menaces againſt himſelf, that
having attempted his life by hanging and
drowning, he would now cut his throat
from ear to ear, if he could burſt through
his reſtrictions, and was in every reſpect
ſo violent and turbulent, with ſo much
dangerous malevolence for the prominent feature of his caſe, that I determined to perſuade his friends to obtain an
order for his admiſſion into a public cha-
rity.

It is to be obſerved, that on the third
day after his being ſent to me, an eruption
of the eryſipetalous kind appeared on his
left arm, with veſications and tumours
of the whole limb, which was ſo much
increaſed by his extraordinary violence,

as

as to produce inflammation and tenfion
of the whole arm from the fhoulder to the
finger ends, that terminated in an abfcefs
above the elbow, which fuppurated and difcharged very profufely. The patient now
began to recover his reafon, and by this
critical difcharge of offending humours,
was entirely reftored to a permanent
ftate of fanity in a few weeks; during
which interval, however, by fome neglect
of his own, or perhaps fome mal-treatment
in thofe who had the fubfequent care of
him, he was deprived of the ufe of his
arm, and has not fince had the free motion of it.

In the two foregoing cafes, it is obvious that the violent efforts of the patients
labouring under a bad habit of body, did
in a great meafure contribute to the pro-
duction of that inflammation which ultimately proved fo falutarily effective.

The fimilitude of effect in both thefe
patients, ferves to fhew how far intemperance and irregularity of living may prove
detrimental to the faculty of reafon;
and how far plethora may be confidered

as

as the immediate caufe of mental derangement; pointing at the fame time the cure
to fuppuration from critical abfcefs, or its
artificial fubftitute of feton or iffue.

C A S E   LXII.

THE records of medicine cannot afford
an inftance fimilar to the prefent, nor do
we find in the different authors who have
profeffedly written on maniacal diforders,
one cafe wherein at fo early a period as
eleven years, the complaint has appeared
with marks fo clear and intelligible.   And
in this inftance it is as fingular, that there
feems to have been no predifpofing caufe
to infanity; no tranflation of difeafed matter to the membranes of the brain, or any
external caufe that could mechanically
operate to produce delirium; no diffufion
of bile, fudden diftention of cutaneous
eruptions, abforption of matter from ab-
fceffes, wounds, or ulcers; no fcrophu-
lous or cancerous ftate of the juices; no
worms,

worms, no deleterious medicine, nor mercurial preparations; no mental caufe; nor
could any hereditary claim be adduced of
the patient's family, either on the father
or mother's fide, having ever been remembered to have been fubject to maniacal affections.   In fact, there was no clue
to direct either to a remote or proximate
caufe of deranged intellect.   This child
was not confidered to poffefs any extraordinary fhare of genius or ability, or re-
marked by activity of imagination; nor
was he fo fprightly as boys of his age generally are, but was rather of a thoughtful
and melancholic difpofition, and very little
inclined to puerile amufements; but on the
whole was tolerably docile and tractable;
had always been healthy, never fhewn a
wanton propenfity to hard and indi-
geftible aliment, nor had in any refpect
been compelled to fuch intenfe or ftudious
application, that could in the leaft affect
his mind.

It was his cuftom to go with other
children to a fchool at fome diftance
from home, and return in the evening.
                                    January

January 29th he came from fchool unufually dull and dejected, but little notice was taken of it then ; but on his return on the following evening, this alteration having vifibly increafed, the caufe
was inquired into, but he could affign no
reafon. And upon the ftricteft examination
it could not be difcovered that he had been
fuddenly frightened, his temper ruffled by
any incident, or that he had undergone the
leaft degree of fcholaftic difcipline or re-
proof. When fpoken to, his anfwers were
vague and inappofite ; he feemed agitated
at the fight of ftrangers ; turned pale and
trembled ; had an angry, acute, ftaring,
look, with dilated pupils, and dreadful apprehenfions that hurried him to examine
every part of the room, as if he expected
to find fome perfon concealed who intended to do him a mifchief. He fometimes appeared timid and diftreffed, fighed, fhed tears, and had not a quarter of an
hour's fleep throughout the night. On
the 31ft, being coftive, fome manna was
diffolved and given, that operated pretty
well,

well, but he ftill continued unufually
ftrange in his manner and actions.   Fear,
diftrefs, and fhame, alternately occupied
his mind; but he could not for a moment fix his attention to any one object.
He was fat up with, but was reftlefs and
had very little fleep.   On the morning of
the firft of February, he fpoke rather more
rationally than on the preceding day, but
complained of a pain in his head, with
vertigo, languor, and dimnefs of fight;
that his eyes ached, and were very painful, and could not tell where he was; he
was laid down to fleep, but was fo reftlefs and diftreffed, he could not procure
the leaft repofe.   If a word was fpoken,
he was peevifh and petulant, and the leaft
motion of any perfon in his prefence rendered him an object of vexation and inquietude.   Being fubject to fhiverings,
and his legs and feet feeling cold, by the
direction of his mother they were foment-
ed with flannels wrung out of warm
water, and he was put to bed again,
when intruding ideas occafioned the fame
per-

pervigilium as before. He frequently
fighed as if labouring under great affliction, was inceffantly talkative, and
rambled from one fubject to another
without the leaft coherence.

February 2nd, the family apothecary
was called in, who found him precifely
in the fame ftate, with alienation of mind,
without fever, the fkin harfh and dry,
fometimes very wakeful and loquacious, at
others ftupid, abfent, and mufing, with the
pulfe rather below the ufual ftandard at
his age. Sinapifms were ufed to his feet,
and a blifter applied to his back. The
night was paffed in a more uneafy and
reftlefs manner than before, and in the
morning, at the particular requeft of the
apothecary, another practitioner was called in, who advifed an emollient warm
fomentation to the belly, thighs, and legs,
and fmall dofes of the pulv. antimonii.
Feb. 3d. His fleep during the night had
been lefs difturbed, but was frequently mingled with fighs and ftartings.
Feb. 4th. All the former figns of mental

tal derangement recurred, and there appeared no alteration for the better. The blifter had difcharged but little. 5th. Had a very reftlefs night. A ftimulative clyfter was inje&ted, but returned again juft tinged with fœces, and was repeated without any favourable effe&t. 6th. Another clyfter anfwered the purpofe, and he appeared tolerably eafy and compofed. The pulv. antimonii was repeated. 8th. He continued alternately in a ftupid or diftrefsfully obftreperous ftate, but at intervals began to evince fome figns of returning reafon, that continued until the 13th, when he relapfed into his former ftate, and having had a miferably reftlefs night, the aggravated fymptoms of diftorted eyes and difficult refpiration increafed his affli&tion. The blifter, that had been rendered perpetual, had difcharged tolerably well; befides which, an iffue was opened in his arm. 15th. An emetic was prefcribed that had no effe&t, and boluffes of camphor and valerian

valerian were adminiftered, but he ftill
continued in the fame aggravated perturbation of mind, without any fever.
17th. Another emetic was given, that
operated tolerably well ; but on the
19th, becoming much worfe in every
refpect, blifters were applied to his legs
by way of revulfion. He had a very bad
night, and was with difficulty kept in bed,
being more irafcible and furious than
at any former period of his illnefs. 20th.
He all day appeared to labour under
the moft poignant fenfations of diftreffed
imagination, and paffed a very bad night.
21ft. The fame fymptoms continued till
towards the morning, when a fullen filence
and referve, accompanied with fome intervals of dofing, fupervened. After fome
hours relaxation he appeared more compofed than he had been for fome time
before, but this was of fhort duration, for
on the 22d he became much worfe, had
fhiverings, with difficulty of breathing,
was furious, and became quite raving, fo
that two very ftout and powerful perfons
could not hold him down in his bed without

great

great exertion.   In this ſtate he continued till the 27th, when immediately after the operation of a laxative medicine, he ſuddenly became more calm and eaſy, and paſſed more water than he had done for ſeveral days before, ſlept with leſs interruption, ſeemed much more rational, and partly recovered his uſual ſpirits.   28th. He reverted into his former ſtate of horror and dejeƈtion, and appeared ſcarcely to know or attend to any external objeƈts.

March 1ſt, he was apparently much leſs diſtreſſed and agitated, and the 3d afforded tranſitory hope that he was getting better, which in ſome meaſure alleviated the painful feelings of maternal affeƈtion, which had ſo long been experienced from an acute ſenſe of his ſufferings ; but this ceſſation of parental ſolicitude was only protraƈted to the 7th, when he appeared again much deranged in his mind, and complained of a pain and weight in the head, which was now direƈted to be ſhaved and bathed with diſtilled vinegar; a bliſter to the occiput was propoſed, as indiſpenſably neceſſary, but the
idea

idea of its application was fo unpleafant
to his friends as to preclude its ufe.   An
emetic much ftronger than any he had before taken, was adminiftered, with no
other effeft than a fmall degree of damp-
nefs upon the fkin.   Hitherto every medical effort had failed, and the poor little
fufferer obtained no permanent relief.
9th. Still a viftim to mercilefs malady,
he was again feized with the moft difmal
apprehenfions and fears; the faculties of
his mind were weak and feeble; taciturnity and meditation fucceeded to horror
and depreffion; fears and lamentations
followed; and as his ruminating paroxyfm
was longer or fhorter, the nights were paffed
with watchfulnefs, and the days in melancholy defpondency, with lucid intervals
of momentary duration, till the 13th,
when the folitary ftate of his mind fuddenly changed into diftraftion, audacity,
and violence.   The delirium appeared to
have taken a turn direftly oppofite to its
former genus; fo that from a ftate of filent defpondency he now became the
raving maniac, and the fituation of him-

felf

felf and family became pitiably deplorable.

At this crifis of calamity a blifter to his
head was popofed, and the former objections being fuperfeded by the emergency
of the cafe, it was applied, and in a few
hours after he became infinitely worfe,
and more raving than before; the caufti-
city of the blifter caufed the moft violent
excitement, and counterbalanced every
benefit that was expected to have occurred from its difcharge : and indeed in a
very long and extenfive practice I never
remember to have feen more than two
inftances of the good effects of vefication
to the head, one of which was in confirmed melancholy, where torpidity and languor had been produced by profufe evacuations ; and the other in a maniacal
affection of fome continuance, where the
powers of nature had been debilitated by
inaction. In the indifcriminate ufe of
epifpaftics for the cure of diforders of the
head, particularly where an over-fulnefs
of the cerebral veffels from the rednefs
and fulnefs of the face, as in phrenitis and

fan-

sanguineous apoplexy, much mischief has been done from their intensely ardent and powerfully stimulating influence. I could recite many instances where blisters applied to the head in furious madness, (in a full habit and sanguine temperament) by increasing the spasmodic stricture, and adding to the excitement of the brain, have proved fatal. 15th. The patient was so very turbulent and restless, that having no strait-waistcoat, and applying no ligatures to his arms and legs, it was with difficulty he was prevented from getting out of bed; in which frantic state he continued till the 17th, on which and the succeeding day other emetics were prescribed, but with no greater efficacy than before. 21st. The violence of the disorder abated, and on that and the ensuing day he was not so loud and raving as before, but often muttered to himself, and appeared stupid, absent, and musing. 23d. He continued much the same, but rather more languid and melancholy, scarcely ever spoke articulately, and remained in that

that ſtate till the 26th, when he ſeemed to recover more of his uſual manner and ſpirits, and was ſuppoſed to be in a ſtate of convaleſcence; but on the 27th, his former mental affections recurring, my advice and aſſiſtance was thought neceſſary, when with all the tender feelings of maternal ſolicitude the preceding detail, which had been carefully committed to paper, was given to me for my peruſal.

The patient had been removed to a remote part of the houſe, and placed in a darkened room, with an aſſiſtant on each ſide of the bed for the purpoſe of coercion. Notwithſtanding the length of his confinement, the violence of his diſorder, and the many viciſſitudes he had experienced, he had neither that morbid nor emaciated appearance that might have been expected. When I approached his bed-ſide, I did not at firſt attract his attention, but after ſpeaking to him, he turned round, and in a deſponding tone of voice, ſaid, "He ſhould never be better, but " that I might do as I pleaſed with him; " that his father was not able to provide
" for

" for him; and that he could not learn
" his book fo well as other boys did."
To which, in a foothing and confoling
manner, I replied, that there was great
probability of doing him good, and getting him quite well, provided my directions were punctually obferved. I appeared by this affurance to have gained
his good opinion, for he fmiled, and
feemed pleafed; and to do my little friend
juftice, when he was himfelf, he never
failed to fecond my endeavours. Perceiving that he often made efforts to leap
out of bed, and that the endeavours of
the attendants to reftrain him only increafed his irritation, I recommended a
ftrait-waiftcoat, which I had brought with
me for that purpofe, and which was occafionally ufed until the completion of the
cure.

From the commencement of the complaint, his appetite had been much depraved. On examination I found fome degree of tenfion and tumour about the epigaftric region, but not accompanied with
any pain, tendernefs, or inflammation.

His

His breath had fometimes been fœtid, but not in the extreme, and was now rather offenfive. His urine had been high-coloured, and was now pale and limpid; but had never been perceived to depofit any fediment, and had been made in fmaller quantities than ufual. Deglutition had been obferved to be more difficult during the paroxyfm of dejeftion, than when in his more delirious ftate; at which times he had always a flight degree of deafnefs, moifture of the eyes, dimnefs of fight, and an involuntary difcharge of tears. He now talked more inconfiftently than when I firft faw him, and complained of ghofts and frightful dreams. When in his moft lucid intervals he appeared ready to fall afleep, had frequent eruftations, and his feet were alternately hot, dry, and cold. His eyes fufficiently indicated the ftate of his mind. The pupils were unufually diftended, and the lids tumid and red, with a fordid rheum adhering to their edges. His face was rather florid, but neither bloated nor fwelled; he expreffed fome childifh fancies,

cies, appeared forgetful, and upon being afked where he felt moft pain, (after two or three times waving his hand, as if in doubt) pointed to his forehead. An equal degree of heat pervaded his whole body, without any apparent augmentation of it in the head and temples. He was naturally difpofed to be coftive; and the ftools which he had had in the courfe of his diforder, when not produced by medicine, were generally hard and high-coloured, and occurred at the intervals of two or three days. He had not the leaft degree of fever, and the functions of his mind were apparently in a deranged ftate. He frequently changed his pofition in bed, with an extraordinary degree of ftrength and agility; and was fo little debilitated, as to retain a greater fhare of mufcular ftrength than is natural to boys in their full health at his age.

I obferved that he appeared to be pleafed at every opportunity he gave his attendants to watch and guard him. His refpiration was entirely free, and he had not any ficknefs at his ftomach. His

fleep

sleep had been much interrupted, and
seldom of long continuance. His sweats
had been partial, chiefly towards the
morning, and seldom continued more
than two minutes; probably from the
restlessness of his body in consequence of
the disturbed state of his mind. In the
paroxysms of mania he had been observed
to grind and gnash his teeth, and had
never appeared thirsty, or to have drank
with eagerness or voracity. His voice
was much lower than its natural extent of
elevation, and he seemed incapable of ar-
ticulating distinctly. His pulse was under sixty, and scarcely perceptible; but
though so weak and low, I considered it a
very fallacious guide, and that it indicated
some obstructions in the heart and lungs,
or an oppression of the cerebellum, and
therefore did not hesitate in performing
the operation of phlebotomy, as the best
preliminary to the completion of the cure.
About six ounces of blood were taken
from the arm; after which the vibration
of the artery was more distinct and accelerated. The blood, when cold, was
covered

covered with a very thin cake of gluten, that adhered to the bason, was bilious, and the ſerum of a yellowiſh complexion. Soon after this operation, he diſcourſed more rationally, and ſeemed leſs drowſy; but in leſs than an hour relapſed into his former ſtate. I directed a ſeton to be made the next morning between the ſcapulæ, in the direction of the ſpine, and that his feet ſhould be immerſed in a warm pediluvium of ſalt and water; and to increaſe perſpiration, that he ſhould often recline his head and face over an earthen veſſel, and inhale the ſteams of hot vinegar, poured upon powdered camphor and the leaves of roſemary; that he ſhould occaſionally be reſtrained by the waiſt-coat, and talked to as little as poſſible. Conſidering the proximate cauſe to occur from a turgeſcency in the cerebral veſſels, I recommended a diet the moſt cooling, ſpare, and ſlender, with almoſt a total abſtinence from liquid food; that drinks of all ſorts ſhould be ſparingly adminiſtered, and in its ſtead roaſted apples, dried cherries, tamarinds, and currant jelly ſhould

be

be prefcribed.   All objects that attract
attention, or excite emotion, were ordered to be removed from his fight, with a
view to keep his mind calm and tranquil ;
fo that all mental irritation being avoided,
the aptitude of frantic paroxyfms might
be diminifhed.   He was ordered to abftain
from all vifcid, flatulent, and grofs food,
and to have at all convenient opportunities more air and exercife.   As emetics
had been fo repeatedly tried without effect,
and might be hazardous, from forcing too
great a quantity of blood to the head, I
objected to their repetition, and prefcribed
a faline purgative mixture, with the foda
phofphorata in an infufion with tincture of
fenna, to be given till fufficient evacuations by ftool fhould be procured, and
occafionally continued.   Having in many
inftances experienced the fedative good
effects of camphor in maniacal diforders, I
adminiftered the following prefcription:

  R Camphora ʒijfs.
   Sp. Vin. R. ʒiij.
    G. Arab. Sacch. Alb. aa ʒij. mifce fimul
denique adde gradatim Aq. Pluvialis fervent. ℥viij.
cujus fumat. Coch. larg. menf. ij. vel iij. ad libitum.

            for

for the form of which I was indebted to
my worthy friend Dr. Rowley, who in his
Treatife on Female and Nervous Difeafes,
judicioufly recommends it as a much better preparation than the julep. e camphor ; becaufe in this the quantity of
the camphor may be better afcertained,
and in the latter it is fo much evaporated
by the ufe of boiling water, as to render
the preparation of doubtful utility, or perhaps in great meafure inefficacious.

28th. The patient paffed a tolerably
eafy night, and had derived the expe&ted
relief from the ufe of the purgative medicine. 29th. He was rather fick at the ftomach: that being attributed to the camphor, it was not given fo often, and in
lefs quantities. 30th. The report was
ftill more favourable; he was rational,
and talked with more recolle&tion and
propriety, but was fubje&t to remitting
pains in his head. 31ft. He was reduced
to as low a ftate, as at the commencement
of his complaint.

April 1. He was tolerably rational, but
complained of his head, with depreffion
of

of fpirits; cried very much, and often
exclaimed that " nobody loved him," and
" he fhould not be happy in another
" world."   2d. He paffed a very indifferent night, was attacked with fhiverings
and yawnings, cried, and evidently laboured under his ufual weight of diftrefs and
anxiety.   The feton began to difcharge
copioufly in the afternoon, his head was
eafier, and he appeared much better.   3d.
Had a tolerably good night, was more
rational and compofed than on the preceding day, and being now confidered in
a convalefcent ftate, there appeared a
probable chance of fuccefs by perfevering
in the mode of cure.   4th. After a tolerable night, was very low and depreffed;
his feet being damp and cold, the warm
pediluvium was repeated : having had
fæcal evacuations on the two or three
preceding days, and the urine having had
its proper courfe, there was no occafion
for aperient medicines.   5th. The functions regular; the difcharge from the feton
was leffened, but from the iffue propor-
tionably increafed.   Slight wanderings
                                    occurred

occurred during the night, but he became more rational in the day-time. This regimen was punctually obferved, and the patient was carried into the open air an hour at a time. 6th. He complained of his belly, was obferved to pick and rub his nofe, with fome degree of lownefs, lofs of voice, palenefs of countenance, complained of naufea at his ftomach, and his breath was unufually fœtid. In the night he was very watchful and incoherent in his expreffions, had troublefome dreams, catching of his lips and eye-lids, with evident fymptoms of indigeftion. 7th. Continued much the fame all day, and in the night was reftlefs and uneafy. The fætor of his breath remaining, rumbling and pricking fenfations of the abdomen, and frequent inclination to ftool, fuggefted the idea of his being afflicted with worms; but as the excrements had never appeared white and flimy, and none had been voided by ftool, their exiftence was a matter of doubt and uncertainty; however, I determined to try the mercur. faccharatus of the Edinburgh difpenfatory,

both

both as a good evacuant and fafe vermifuge; after being twice given, it occafioned three dejections in the fpace of a
few hours, but no worms, or any thing of a
verminous nature appearing in the ftools,
and the fymptoms that had given rife to this
fufpicion ftill continuing, the more effectually to diflodge them, if they did actually exift, one grain of the gum. gutt.
gambog. with half a grain of calomel, and
a fcruple of facchar. alb. made into a
powder, were exhibited at proper intervals; befides which fome garlic, cut fmall,
was given in warm milk, but neither producing the leaft appearance of worms, and
the patient being apparently worfe in
many refpects than before thefe medicines
were given, he returned to his ufual
medicines and regimen. The purgatives
being intermitted as ufual, he had at
this æra a partial fuppreffion of urine,
which was foon removed by mild diu-
retics.

An obfervation was made, that he
was moft in his fenfes, and his head
always cleareft, when he paffed moft

water,

water, and that this had invariably been the cafe fince the commencement of his diforder. It was therefore a fymptom that required more particular attention; and for the promotion of which, fp. nitr. d. in parfley-root tea, with the warm pedi-luvium, greatly contributed.   12th. He appeared in every refpect much better, his mind was quiet and collected, he was taken into the air, and paffed the day in a much more rational manner than at any former period of the complaint, but in the evening became very low, fighed, and was incongruous in his fpeech and behaviour, but not turbulent; flept little that night, and the next morning ap-peared drowfy and low fpirited, which was in great meafure attributed to his having taken cold in his airing the day before.   13th. After having had a toler-ably good night, he got up and dreffed himfelf, walked about the room, and was very rational.   The feton, which had been very fore and painful, difcharged more copioufly, and became eafier. Hav-ing had no ftool for two days, the purga-

T   tive

tive medicine was given, and repeated at proper diſtances ; but not having had its uſual effeɛt, in the evening an emollient clyſter was adminiſtered, that produced ſtools of a fœtid nature.   This night his perſpiration was more general, and of longer continuance than at any former period of his illneſs ; but he was watchful and reſtleſs.   14th. He was very ſenſible, and at his own requeſt was again taken into the air, where he remained ſome hours, and continued tolerably rational all day, but in the evening was depreſſed and low, with ſlight wanderings, and complained of pain and weight in his head.   The warm pe-diluvium was made uſe of for half an hour before, and at bed-time the camphorated mixture was given, but his ſleep was diſturb-ed with terrifying dreams ; he had no ſtool, and in the morning awoke very ſorrow-ful and dejeɛted, and continued ſo through-out the greateſt part of the day. 15th. Con-tinued much the ſame; in the forenoon the camphorated mixture was adminiſter-ed, and in the afternoon the purgative medicine, that produced no effeɛt ; he had

little

little or no appetite, appeared to be out
of temper, and at intervals talked wild
and inconfiftently.   In the evening an
emollient clyfter was given, without effect.
The night was paffed with watchfulnefs,
and his fleep was interrupted with frightful dreams. 16th. Appeared much clearer
in his intellects, but complained of pain
in his head, with tenfion of the abdomen,
and difficult refpiration. The ol. ricini
was prefcribed inftead of the former purgative; the fecond dofe of which procured
a ftool foon after it was taken, but he had
not paffed any water for the laft twenty-
four hours. The fp. nitr. d. was therefore again adminiftered in parfley-root
tea, and repeated until the defired purpofe was accomplifhed ; he continued
calm all the day, though not very rational, and had a better night than before.
17th. Was very low, converfed but little,
and was at times incoherent in his actions
and behaviour ; continued fo all day, and
had a very indifferent night. 18th. Had
a free paffage, and had no occafion for

either

either the drops or oil.   19th. Was calm
and confiftent; his feet, from the ufe of
the warm pediluvium, continued moift
and warm; he perfpired during his fleep,
which was longer and lefs interrupted;
the urine was made freely, appeared of
a red colour, and depofited a light fediment.   20th. He continued in a comfortable ftate, had a very good night, and his
appetite returned. On the 21ft was very low,
complained of a pain in his head; and not
having had a ftool for three days, a fpoon-
ful of the ol. ricini was repeated, that anfwered the purpofe foon after it was given,
and relieved his head; he remained cool
and rational during the day, and had a
very good night.   22d. At his own requeft, he was feated in a carriage, and
drawn about in the open air for feveral hours, and indulged in any little amufement he defired, but with the admonitory
precaution that he fhould not dwell too
long on any particular objeft.   He now
began to fpeak and amufe himfelf in his
ufual manner, and with more vivacity
than

than before his diforder occurred; he
wifhed to ride on horfeback, but which at
prefent was thought improper.

As the fingularity of his cafe had excited fome degree of curiofity, many perfons had a defire to fee him; of whom
none were admitted but thofe who had
previoufly been his familiar acquaintance.
And when he faw any ftranger, it was re-
marked, that it did not hurry or agitate
him fo much as might have been expected
from the weak ftate of his mind. He
continued under the fame regulation of
diet and medicine, in a quiet and rational
ftate, till the 10th of May, when after an
indifferent night he was early in the morning attacked with his former dejection,
and his mind became alternately agitated
with fear, forrow, fufpicion, and folitude,
and he continued fo during that day.
Having had no regular ftool for two days,
the ol. ricini was repeated, and the firft
dofe produced no effect, but the fecond
was attended with better fuccefs. From
this, and fome fleep that he procured in
the former part of the night, he received
but

but little benefit. The pediluvium and camphorated mixture were continued regularly. 12th. He became more tranquil, but complained of pain in the lower part of his bowels, that was removed by a ftimulating clyfter, after two dofes of the oil had been given in vain, 13th. He was afflicted with a violent pain in the fore part of his head, and his eyes being flightly inflamed, with the lids fwelled and very red, by my direction a furgeon was fent for to bleed him, who objected to the operation, from the low ftate of his pulfe; but at the requeft of his mother, and from refpect to my advice, the opinion was over-ruled, and he took away eight ounces of blood. He bled very freely, and did not experience any lofs until his arm was binding up, when he turned pale, his lips became white, and he perfpired all over, but recovered without fainting. The pulfe, after bleeding, as in the former cafe, was obferved to rife, become ftronger, and more accelerated. Upon inquiry I found the blood of a flight buffy appearance; which being divided

vided and put into fcales, the craffamen-
tum weighed three ounces and three
quarters, and the ferum nearly five ounces;
which experiment was made at the requeft and for the fatisfaction of his mother. The feton had difcharged but little, and the iffue confiderably; an alter-
native that had been before obferved.
After bleeding, he paffed a good night,
and was tolerably well all the next day.

15th. Was rather dull and penfive,
and was not fo rational and confiftent in
his converfation. Having had no ftool,
the oil was repeated without effect; a third
dofe, however, anfwered the purpofe.
16th. Was more clear and confiftent. 17th. Very dull and unwilling to
fpeak, or be fpoken to, and feemed to
attend very little to external objects.
Having made no water the former day
and night, it was obtained as ufual by the
nitre drops and tea. 18th. Having had
a very good night, and a natural ftool in
the morning, he appeared much better in
every refpect, and was throughout the
whole day more rational, ftill, and tractable.

able. 19th. He appeared quite comfortable, obvioufly in a ftate of convalefcence,
and defired that he might ride on horfeback. To this I affented, and defired at
the fame time that he might receive every
admiffible gratification.

From this period he remained rational
in his converfation, and confiftent in his
behaviour, but fometimes too high-fpi-
rited, and rather ungovernable; and without the interpofition of fome authority, he
was not eafily prevailed upon to perfevere
in a neceffary regimen; for having re-
gained his liberty, and experiencing the
indulgent partiality naturally refulting
from parental pleafure at his recovery,
he began to be impatient of reftraint, although upon the whole he had conformed
as well to order as could reafonably be
expected. A fudden flight inflammation
occurring in his right eye, it was thought
neceffary to repeat the bleeding on the
7th of June, from which æra his progrefs
to convalefcence was remarkably rapid,
and he continued uninterruptedly in poffeffion of his mental faculties, to the comfort

fort and fatisfaction of his friends and
relatives. The feton was healed up
a few days after the laft bleeding, but
the iffue was continued open. It is
truly fingular, that fince his recovery
his temper and difpofition have regene-
rated, without the leaft veftige of that
referve and dulnefs which had always
before been the prominent traits of his
character *.

CASE

* Sorry, Loco citat. 2 part, cap. 3. p. 284. mentions,
that he himfelf knew a cafe of a child having been abfolutely *born mad*. A woman of about forty years of
age, of a full and plethoric habit of body, who conftantly laughed and did the ftrangeft things, but who
independently of thefe circumftances enjoyed the very
beft health, fell about twelve or fourteen years ago,
after a fevere and tedious labour, in which fhe was
delivered of a daughter, into a very great weaknefs of
underftanding. This gradually increafed, and during
the laft war fhe one day entered the foreft with her
daughter, and deftroyed her in a fhocking manner.
A fhort time before her hufband's death, fhe became
pregnant, and on the 20th of January 1763, was brought
to bed without any affiftance, of a male child who was
raving mad. When he was brought to our workhoufe,
which was on the 24th, he poffeffed fo much ftrength
in his legs and arms, that four women could at times
with difficulty reftrain him. Thefe periods either
ended

CASE LXIII.

A Man, about forty-eight years of age, of a gloomy difpofition, and melancholy temperament; without any apparent caufe, on a fudden became fullen, referved, irafcible, and morofe, and fhewed a great propenfity to fuicide; his mind gradually funk into the moft diftrefsful ftate of melancholy and deje&ion: his memory was very defe&ive, his fleep was interrupted, his lucid intervals were of fhort and momentary duration, his appetite was depraved, there was a ftubborn conftipation of the bowels: he was fometimes very deaf; fubje&t to eru&ations with involuntary motions of the eyes; the countenance was pallid, bloated, and fwelled; the fkin harfh and

ended with indefcribable laughter, for which no evident reafon could be obferved, or elfe he tore in anger every thing near him, clothes, linen, bed furniture, and every thread he could get hold of; and we durft not leave him alone, or he would get on the tables and benches, and even attempt to climb up the walls; afterwards, however, when he began to have teeth, he fell into a general wafting, or decline, and died!

dry;

dry; he was feized with the moft ridiculous fears and apprehenfions, and now
and then complained of a pain, which he
faid refembled what he thought he fhould
have felt if a nail had been driven into his
head; uneafinefs in the right hypochondrium, that upon examination was found
rather hard and fwelled.

He had taken feveral vomits, and had
a blifter to his head, without deriving the
leaft advantage from either. He had
never been in the leaft reftrained from
fluids, but on the contrary was fuffered to
indulge in the free ufe of them; but in
particular of thofe to which he was moft
partial. His pulfe in general was about
eighty, rather weak and fmall to the touch,
but rofe higher after bleeding. Cathartics
were occafionally adminiftered: a feton
was paffed between his fhoulders in the
direction of the fpine, and ten grains of
camphor, in the form of a bolus, were
given four times a day. Abftinence from
fluids was obferved with the ftricteft care
and circumfpection; their quantity being
gradually diminifhed, and almoft totally
left

left off at the expiration of five months.
At this æra there remained little or no
incongruity of idea : his perceptions became clear, and his judgment as found as
at any former period of his life.   He vo-
luntarily remained with me fome months
after the cure was completed, and has
ever fince retained the full enjoyment of
his health and reafon.

────────────

C A S E   LXIV.

M. C. a young lady about the age of
twenty-feven, of a habit obnoxious to inflammatory diforders, whofe mother had
been feveral times infane, and frequently
under my care, was fuddenly feized with a
rigor, that was fucceeded by an acute inflammatory fever, a quick, full, and tenfe
pulfe, great heat and thirft, and pains in
the head, back, or loins, with flight delirium, giddinefs, and dimnefs of fight.   To
moderate the febrile fymptoms, venefection,
cooling diaphoretics, and diluting drinks
were

were prescribed. On the ninth day succeeding the attack loose stools and turbid
urine confirmed the crisis of the disorder.
The cortex took place as a tonic, and she
was thought to be in a promising state of
convalescence, but anxiety and solicitude
of mind very unusual to her before this
illness, supervening, confirmed her friends
that she possessed the morbid inheritance
of her mother. Her appetite was depraved, her pulse quick and hard, her
breath uncommonly hot and offensive, she
talked wild, with almost incessant vociferation; obtained little sleep, and less per-
spiration; frequently described images that
had no existence but in her own idea:
often shuddered with cold, and afterwards
became hot and thirsty.

After continuing in this state several
days, she was committed to my care. I
found she had been suffered to drink co-
piously of diluting liquors; the eye-lids
were red, puffed, and tumid; the tunica
albuginea was inflamed, and the pupils
were much distended; there was a flori-
dity in her face that approached to the
gutta

gutta rofacea; the tongue was much dif-
coloured, and fhe had a difficulty in refpiration.   At intervals fhe became filent,
referved, and melancholy, and at other
times was fo obftreperous and violent, as
to oblige thofe who had the care of her to
have recourfe to coercive meafures; the
pulfe was hard, and chord-like, and at an
hundred and twenty in a minute. *Venæ-
fectio ad deliquium* was advifed; the blood
was in a very inflamed ftate : neutral falts
were occafionally adminiftered, and the
warm pediluvium was ufed every night
before fhe went to bed; the camphorated
mixture with nitre was given at ftated intervals, and abftinence from fluids as much
as poffible enjoined for nearly two months,
in which time, venefection being thrice
repeated, the mental perturbation that was
evidently dependent on the fever, and a
type thereof, together with the primary
caufe, had a favourable termination. She
continued with me a confiderable time
after the cure, and had no relapfe, and
has ever fince continued well in her intellects.

The

The advantage refulting from abfti-nence from fluids, in too great a turgency of the cerebral veffels, is fufficiently obvi-ous in the three preceding cafes, and many more might be introduced to con-firm the propriety of adhering to fuch a practice; but the injunction is of fo fevere and unpleafant a nature, and felf-denial fo difficult, that it feldom happens that patients have fufficient refolution and per-feverance to accede to a regular confor-mity thereto; and it is too often neglected by thofe who have the care of maniacs, in thofe cafes where it might be adopted with the happieft profpect of fuccefs.

CASE LXV.

THE well-written letter, defcriptive of this patient's cafe, is literally tranfcribed as follows:

" Auguft 30th, 1778.
" SIR,
" Your favour of the 4th inftant I re-ceived, and fhould have anfwered it be-fore,

fore, but waited to give you the prefent fymptoms. The perfon I wrote to you about, is a young man of twenty-eight years of age, of a delicate, thin conftitution. It will be fix years next Chriftmas fince he was bit by a dog. It was fancied the dog was mad, but many perfons having been bit by the fame dog, who took no farther notice of it, and no ill confequence following it, confirms the dog not being mad. This young man was advifed to be dipt in the fea, and take fome medicines as preventives, the chief ingredients of which were native and factitious cinnabar. He took thefe medicines fo long, till he found himfelf much weakened by them, and has frequently complained fince of a giddinefs in his head, and a relaxation at times laft fummer. He almoft every evening ufed moft violent exercife at fives. As we impute his prefent diforder to thefe caufes, I thought it proper to mention them, though we never obferved any thing remarkable in him till the fixth or feventh of October laft. He had been a few days on a journey on bufinefs. The evening he returned he appeared to be in an odd

whimfical

whimfical way, and being inconfiftent in converfation, which was imputed to his being in liquor, and no notice being taken of it, he went to bed, prefently rofe again, and infifted on going out. The fervants let him out. He remained out all night in the fields in a hard rain. The next morning he returned and complained of a moft violent pain in his head, and that he had not flept fince his leaving home; was very feverifh and unaccountably whimfical. Fancied he had been poifoned, and that every thing that was offered him was impregnated with poifon. He complained of violent and acute pains in his head for half an hour together, when the pain ceafed, it left an odd fenfation like the crawling of fomething within-infide the fkin. Sometimes exceeding ftrong, then faint and weak, fmelt difagreeable fmells, was exceeding timorous, had violent flufhings, then deadly palenefs fucceeded. At his firft feizure he had no appetite, then a moft extraordinary one. Sudden gufts of paffion, with ftrong averfions and affections to different objects. Violent

u   convulfive

convulfive motions in his arms and legs, frequent and deep fighings ; his water limpid, with a fediment like fand ; fometimes a great thirft.

" He found no relief from any thing but blifters on his legs, which were kept open till a mortification was apprehended, and drinking ftrong mutton broth frequently about Chriftmas he grew better, and has been able to follow his bufinefs, though not perfectly well. As he has always been low, and rather fhewed an averfion to converfation or cheerfulnefs, fince then we have obferved him peculiarly low, between the laft quarter and firft of the moon, at which time he has from the firft appeared moft affected. About two months ago he went to fpend a few days with a friend by the fea. He drank rather more than his ufual quantity, which has not exceeded three or four glaffes of beer and wine after dinner and fupper fince his firft illnefs. The next morning he rofe early and bathed. At breakfaft he complained of great pain in his head, and that he had not flept all night, and was very feverifh

Within thefe few days he feems a little cheerful for a fmall fpace of time. He has a very great averfion to converfation, and generally a very great languor and relaxation, attended with numbnefs and flight pains at particular parts. Till laft Thurfday, he has taken very little, fince which he begins to recover his appetite. For fome time he has been perfuaded to drink valerian tea, with feven drops of acid elixir of vitriol. At the beginning of his illnefs he had an iffue cut in his arm, which difcharged greatly, but about fix or feven weeks ago he had it dried up. And in vain hitherto has he been entreated to have another. We are fometimes afraid his fenfes will be loft in childifhnefs; at others have great hopes: but as his complaint varies fo often, we can form no opinion of him. The roots of his nails have frequently turned black. He has grown moft exceedingly thin, and by nature was never robuft. For thefe two months he has drank nothing but fmall beer and water, and lived very low. We

are

are the more anxious for him, as he has nothing but his bufinefs to depend on, which muft fail if he has no relief : but pleafe God to reftore him. He is in a genteel way; I therefore hope you will confider his cafe, and do your beft for him. I flatter myfelf you are capable. You will let me know your fee, that it may be remitted you at the time when you fend your prefcription. Beg you will acquaint me what regimen he ought to follow, and how he fhould be treated, as hitherto he has always been indulged in his whims. I am, Sir,

"Your refpectful humble fervant."

In confequence of the above applica-tion, iffues were directed to be opened in the left arm betwixt the biceps and del-toid mufcles, and in the interior part of the leg in the fame fide, in the cavity be-low the knee. The vegetable bitters were prefcribed, with the camphorated mixture, and an agglutinating regimen. The ufe of the cold bath, and gentle coercion, as occafion

occafion might require.   By which means
the diforder was mitigated, and the patient
enabled to purfue his wonted avocations.

CASE   LXVI.

INSANITY having for many years been
the immediate object of the author's practice, he may venture to affirm, that of
every fpecies of madnefs, that which is
occafioned by religious enthufiafm is by
far the moft difficult of cure, and oftener
than any other proves the fource of
defpair, which terminates in fuicide.

G. L. aged forty-eight, having an hereditary difpofition to melancholy, for a
confiderable time endured many troublefome and vexatious cares and difappoint-
ments in life, which he had encountered
with all poffible fortitude ; at length the
accumulated affliction of lofing a valuable
relation, caufed him to fink into a low and
defponding ftate of mind, when unfortunately becoming acquainted with a gloomy
fanatic

fanatic teacher of the methodiftical order,
his mind being but too well prepared
to imbibe the poifonous tenets of his doctrine, he foon became enthufiaftically mad.
When I was introduced to him, to ufe the
words of a celebrated poet,

" He wore affliction in his afpect,
" And the black cloud that lour'd on his brow,
" Seem'd to declare ftrange wretchednefs of forrow."

His anxiety was extreme; he had an even
regular pulfe, but feldom any appetite;
was obftinately coftive; flept little, and
perfpired lefs; he was fubject to fugitive palenefs; the urine was copious and
coloured; and his tafte and fmell were
much impaired: overwhelmed with religious defpondency, he entertained confufed ideas of the terrors, rewards, and
punifhments of a future life; believed he
was forfaken of the Almighty, and was
become an object of his wrath, and was
doomed to condign punifhment. It was
in vain to argue with him. Emetics were
adminiftered; the camphorated mixture,
and the warm pediluvium fucceeded; a
fèton

feton for a confiderable time was kept
open in the back, but all proved ineffectual. He remained a victim to defpair,
fecluded from fociety; and it required
Cerberian vigilance to prevent his termi-
nating his own exiftence, that concluded
in a pulmonary confumption, which occurred in the fifty-fecond year of his age.

CASE LXVII.

In October 1791, I was defired to vifit
a gentleman of great refpectability, whofe
intellectual faculties were much impaired
by too clofe an application to religious
enthufiafm. From a pleafant, lively, focial companion, he had degenerated into a
morofe, fullen, and referved reclufe: that
courtefy, once fo amiable in his manners
and addrefs, were now no longer confpicuous; his whole fyftem was impregnated
with the poifon of methodifm; its doctri
nal terrors had reduced him to the loweft
ebb of melancholy and defpair; he derived

rived no relief whatever from medical advice and regimen, nor would he attend to any reafonable remonftrances from his friends, but gave himfelf up for loft. His thoughts were fo invincibly determined on fuicide, that he had nearly effected his own deftruction in feveral attempts, and the greateft care and precaution were not fufficient ultimately to prevent that fatal cataftrophe.

CASE LXVIII.

IN this cafe of a married lady, aged thirty, there was no difpofition to infanity, previous to the pretended miraculous interpofition of one of thofe itinerant fanatics, whofe aim is to cloud and wound the feelings of their profelytes; fhe was taught to believe that fhe actually committed fins of which fhe had fcarcely the leaft conception, and to ufe her own expreffion, that " fhe was inevitably loft to falvation." Being naturally felf-willed and impatient, the good counfel, remonftrances, and admonitions

monitions of her friends proved ineffectual: the mifery of her mind counterbalanced every confideration of the prefent and future advantage of life, and fhe
formed a determined refolution to deftroy
that exiftence which, through internal anguifh and horror, was become infupportable: being determined to complete this
crime, having deeply engraven with a
fharp-pointed inftrument on her left arm,
her chriftian and furname, the day of the
month, date of the year, and place of her
abode, for the direct purpofe, as fhe declared to me, of being owned when found,
fhe fuddenly eloped from her home, with
an intent to drown herfelf in a river not
far diftant; but being purfued and brought
back by her friends, it was determined to
place her in an houfe appointed for the
reception of lunatics, where, notwithftanding every poffible means were ufed,
that medicine or humanity could effect,
or caution devife, fuch was her devoted
purpofe, that fhe effected it in a manner
that would appear incredulous to thofe
who are unacquainted with the almoft

fuper-

fupernatural cunning and contrivance attached to dementated human nature.

CASE LXIX.

THIS patient had been bred to the
law, but having a fufficiency, independent
of his profeffion, declined that practice.
He was by nature a humourift, and poffeffing a lively imagination, frequented convivial meetings, in which focieties he was
efteemed a *bon vivant*. In this courfe of
life he accidentally formed an acquaintance
with a perfon who had been deluded into
falfe notions of religion, by one of thofe
itinerant preachers with which this country unfortunately abounds: he inftanta-
neoufly imbibed thofe poifonous doctrines,
and as if by a charm, became fo infatuated
as to avoid his former acquaintance, abo-
lifh every focial pleafure, prefer folitude,
and to confider his eternal fate as irre-
deemable : the Supreme Being had been
reprefented to him as partial and vindictive,

and

and delighting in the punifhment of his creatures, which caufed his ideas to be overwhelmed with melancholy and dejeƈtion: for a confiderable time he laboured under the moft painful mortification of both body and mind, and having more than once attempted his own life, his friends thought it indifpenfably neceffary to remove him to a place appropriate to his unhappy fituation, where I was requefted to vifit and prefcribe for him; he appeared much emaciated, reftlefs, averfe to converfation, and loft in thought, and when approached, was timid and fufpicious. He had a fufco-pallid complexion, little fleep of nights, and wept and fighed inceffantly: in this diftrefsful fituation he continued feveral months, and rejeƈted all medical advice and affiftance: but not being able any longer to refift the means of relief, a feton was paffed between the fhoulders in the direƈtion of the fpine, and antimonial emetics were repeated every fourth or fifth evening; in the day he took the camphorated mixture, and again at night with the addition of tinƈtura fuliginis, and the oleum ricini as an occafional laxative.

laxative. His officious friend and adviser was prevented from feeing him, and a worthy clergyman of his acquaintance undertook the benevolent and humane task of administering that spiritual confolation that was requisite ; which with a regular adherence to medical assistance, in two months restored him to that state of convalescence, which, not being disturbed by any relapse, ultimately brought him to a due sense of rectitude and religion.

CASE LXX.

Mr. W. M. aged thirty-eight, who had long fulfilled the duties of a private life with credit to himself and advantage to his family, by contracting an acquaintance with a travelling paftor, who made it his bufinefs to disseminate the doctrine of the methodists, and who had bewildered his imagination with dreadful ideas of a vindictive Deity, and the punishments of an eternal state, suddenly became much altered in his conduct and behaviour :
fometimes

fometimes he was fo much depreffed in
mind as to lock himfelf up in a room for
whole days together, and would not fpeak
to any perfon ; at others his paffions
would be inflamed to fuch a degree of
provocation as to caufe him to threaten
the lives of thofe about him. At others
he would inceffantly talk in a confufed
manner on religious fubjects, and defpairing of forgivenefs in a future ftate, declared his intention of deftroying himfelf,
which he would certainly have effected,
had not the greateft care been taken to
prevent him. Being thus incapable of
conducting his bufinefs with his cuftomary
order and regularity, his friends thought
it proper to place him under my care.
By undergoing a treatment nearly fimilar
to that inferted in the preceding cafe, with
this difference, that an iffue in his arm
that had been neglected and dried up
during his derangement, was re-opened;
in fome confiderable time he recovered
his reafon, and was able to return home,
and by avoiding the company and converfation of the malevolent miffionary, to
whofe

whose religious delufions he had before fallen a prey, has fince continued to conduct himfelf with propriety, and remained free from maniacal affection.

We are indebted to the ingenious Dr. Pargeter, for the following inftances of that fpecies of mania that originates from religious enthufiafm. He was fent for to a refpectable farmer in the country, whom he found very low and melancholy, inconfiftent in his converfation, and feeming to labour under great diftrefs concerning his future ftate. His friends had before been obliged to place him in a houfe appropriated for the reception of lunatics. He could render him very little fervice, as he was unable to remove the caufe of his complaint : the patient's misfortunes he relates to have originated in a very curious circumftance. He was publicly reproved for fleeping during divine fervice by a clergyman, which gave him fo much offence, that he feceded from the church, and attached himfelf to the methodifts, by whom he was reduced to the unhappy ftate in which he found him :

he

he could not, on the ftricteft inquiry learn,
that previous to this circumftance he had
exhibited any fymptoms of mental derangement, but was efteemed a very pleafant and cheerful companion. He was
defired to vifit a woman, who refided at
no great diftance from the former patient,
whom he found fitting up in bed, with cloaks
and flannels wrapped round her head,
neck, and fhoulders. She received him
with a fmiling countenance, and when he
inquired into the caufe and nature of her
complaints, fhe laughed, and enumerated
a great variety of fymptoms, but he could
not difcover that fhe had any bodily indifpofition. In a chair by the bed-fide
were Wefley's Journal, Watts's Hymns,
the Pilgrim's Progrefs, and the Fiery Fur-
nace of Affliction. He prefcribed according to the ufual form, but could render her no fervice, and was informed that
fhe afterwards became fo mad as to require
clofe confinement. Her hufband acquainted him, that before this attack fhe
had not the leaft predifpofition to infanity;
and it appeared that a methodift preacher,

x   who

who had much infefted the parifh, was frequently in her company, and they were perpetually converfing on religious fub-jects. He alfo adds, that he attended a young woman with a peripneumony, oc-cafioned by fome tea, or bread and butter paffing down the trachea in a fit of laugh-ter. As the fymptoms were acute and fufpicious, he paid more than ordinary attention to her cafe, vifiting her twice, and often three times in a day; he fcarcely ever went into her room, but he faw a man with a book in his hand, whom he afterwards learned was a methodift. One day when he called, the girl was exclaim-ing " Oh fweet Chrift! Dear Chrift! I " do love Chrift!" He afked her what fhe meant. She told him fhe had feen and had been talking to her dear Chrift. The patient fortunately loft her complaint, and being enabled to return to her former occupa-tions, her mind was gradually weaned from thofe delufions, which might proba-bly have terminated in confirmed mania. He obferves, that the advantage which this fanatic took of this girl's ignorance

and

and indifpofition, might not improperly
be compared to the conduct of thofe
wretches, who by availing themfelves of
the confufion of a fire, plunder the unhappy fufferers. And adds, that the pre-
valence of methodifm, with its deplorable
effects in the neighbourhood where this
girl refided, might, he fays, be afcribed to
an opulent tradefman, who maintained a
preacher in the capacity of a domeftic
chaplain, who was a failor in the laft war.
He was one day haranguing on the fubject of hell-flames, and took occafion to
obferve that he could not give a defcription adequate to the horrors of that place,
although he had been there *eleven months:*
a wag, whom curiofity had induced to
liften to him, called out, " I wifh you had
" ftaid there another month, and then you
" would have gained a fettlement." Our
author further remarks, that fuch infatua-
tion is the more melancholy, as it tends to
augment the number of fuicides in a na-
tion, that is fuppofed to be more generally addicted to that crime than any
other in Europe, which has caufed the

French

French to adopt our word *fuicide* into their language as an *Anglicifm*. Such confequences, however, from this particular caufe, muft convince all perfons of a found underftanding, of the errors of thofe tenets which caufe or very greatly conduce to it, fince genuine Chriftianity muft very powerfully deter men from this unnatural violence.

CASE LXXI.

JOHN UPTON, (on the 29th of Auguft 1792,) a labouring man, who for fome time had fhewn fymptoms of infanity, and whofe mind had been previoufly worked upon by miftaken zealots, even to religious frenzy, conceived a refolution of deftroying himfelf and family, which he unhappily perpetrated. A neighbour going early into the yard, difcovered his wife dead on the fteps, her head and body fhockingly beaten and bruifed; and on further fearch a youth was found under a table, with his head beaten to a mummy; and

and in the garret this miferable wretch was found fufpended, who had attempted to put a period to his exiftence with a knife; but not having refolution to cut his throat, he effeéted his diabolical purpofe by hanging himfelf.

CASE LXXII.

AN elderly woman, who refided in the neighbourhood of Bifhop's Auckland, and had for fome years been reduced to extreme poverty, on the firft news of her becoming poffeffed of a large fortune, became unufually dull and penfive. This was fucceeded by a profound taciturnity and objeétion to all kinds of fuftenance. She would lament, weep, and figh, as if fome weighty misfortune had befallen her. At length, when fhe was nearly ftarved, it was difcovered that fhe had eaten fome food that was left in her apartment for that purpofe, of which no notice was taken. The food that was fupplied from

this

this æra, was regularly eaten. In Auguſt
1790, ſhe was taken to London. She
had a very morbid countenance, with
permanent paleneſs, impreſſed with a fixed
ſullenneſs and downcaſt looks ; and notwithſtanding every medical effort was
exerted towards her relief, ſhe continued
in this melancholy ſtate until the December following, when a general atrophy
cauſed her death. From this, and many
other inſtances, it is obvious how very injurious are the exceſſive tumults of ſudden
joy and proſperity, both to body and
mind.

The following is another inſtance of
the truth of the above aſſertion. A man,
who lived among the miſcreants of Saint
Giles's, by iſſue of a legal proceſs was
found to be a principal proprietor of
Brompton-Row, and other valuable pre-
miſes, to the amount of £30,000, This
ſudden tranſition of fortune operated ſo
unfortunately on his mind, that he inſtantly became inſane, and has continued
ſo ever ſince. Hence it may be inferred,
that misfortune being the lot of mankind,

it

it requires greater ftrength of intellectual powers to moderate and refift the intoxicating effects of fudden profperity, than to repel the moft powerful attacks of adverfity.

Here it is not improper to remark, that the celebrated Dr. Mead, upon the authority of Dr. Hall, who was at that time phyfician to Bethlem-Hofpital, obferves, that among the number of perfons who became infane in confequence of their connexion with the South-Sea-Company, in the year 1723, there was a much larger proportion of thofe fuccefsful adventurers, whom fortune had favoured with a fudden acquifition of immenfe riches, than of thofe who were completely ruined by that iniquitous impofition.

CASE LXXIII.

T. M. a farmer, whofe refidence was in the Weald of Kent, who for fome months had been placed under my care, was often

vifited

vifited by his friends, with whom he converfed in fo rational a manner, that contrary to my advice they thought proper
to agree to his folicitations, and permit him
to return home, which he did in a few
days. For fome time he behaved in fuch
a manner as to juftify the meafure, and to
caufe fome regret that they had not
fooner complied with his wifhes. But
the futility of this opinion was proved
by his fuddenly committing an act of
defperation, that put a period to his exiftence in a few days after his return home.

Many other inftances might be fub-
joined of the improper liberation of lunatics, many of which have occurred in my
own practice; but I fhall content myfelf
with this obfervation, that the lucid intervals which occur to the unhappy victims of
infanity, have fometimes been of fo long
duration, as to induce a general idea of
their complete recovery, and felect a few
cafes as neceffary precautions to thofe
who have the difpofal of fuch unhappy
perfons, to act with caution and mature
deliberation, before they are prevailed on to
liften

liften ferioufly to their artful infinuations, or comply with their infidious requefts.

A young gentleman afflicted with this melancholy infirmity, lately appeared to all his friends fo entirely recovered, that his liberation was generally agreed on; but juft as he was quitting the refidence where he had remained for a confiderable time, he begged to return for a moment, as he had a very particular letter to difpatch to the Holy Ghoft, which by his friends was thought fuch fufficient proof of lunacy as to induce them to continue him in *ftatu quo.*

In the year 1788, as the Rev. William Norman, Rector of Bledan, in the county of Somerfet, was fitting at fupper with a friend, he obferved his brother, the Rev. Henry Norman, take a large knife from the cafe, and go into the kitchen. He immediately called to the fervants to take it from him, which through fear they omitted to do. Soon after Henry returned to the parlour with the knife concealed under his coat, and unobferved by his brother, came behind him and ftabbed him twice. The unfortunate gentleman
lay

lay in the greatest agonies of pain till
Sunday morning, when he expired.   The
wretched perpetrator of this horrid deed
was rector of a parish near Winchester,
and having been some time before deranged in his intellects, was removed to
his brother's at Bledan for security, where
for a confiderable time together he behaved in a more ferene state than for some
years before, and had a greater share of
liberty allowed him, which ended in the
tragical manner above related.

In January 1791, a poor woman much
deranged in her intellects, who had been
confined in the workhoufe at Sheffield
a confiderable time, but was thought
fo fufficiently recovered as to be able
to return home to her hufband, after continuing three weeks without any vifible
return of her diforder, fhe threw her child,
an infant about three weeks old, into the
river Sheaf near the bridge at that place,
and a great stone after it.   Providentially
a man was paffing over the bridge, and
feeing fomething struggling in the water,
he afked the unhappy woman what fhe had
thrown

thrown in? fhe exultingly anfwered, Her
child.   The man, with a warmth of humanity that did him credit, inftantly
jumped off the bridge, and precipitated
himfelf into the water, by which he was
confiderably hurt, but prevented the babe
from perifhing.   It had not received any
material injury, and was foon perfectly
recovered.   The mother was remanded
to her former confinement.

A perfon named Childs, who had for
a long time obtained his livelihood by attending on infane perfons in different
parts of Chefhire, was employed a few
years fince to take care of a gentleman
who refided near Namptwich.   Having
from long experience derived fome knowledge of thefe unfortunate cafes, the patient was principally left to the care of
Childs; and after fome time, every fymptom appearing to demonftrate the return
of reafon, he whilft in this evidently amend-
ing ftate, was treated with an increafed
degree of indulgence.   He one day requefted that his keeper would entruft him
with a razor to fhave himfelf.   The man

at

at firſt peremptorily refuſed, but by the rational entreaties of the patient was at length induced to give a reluctant conſent, and conſequently provided him with the neceſſary apparatus. He accordingly ſat down before the glaſs, and having ſhaved one ſide of his face, called his keeper to ſee with what dexterity he had partly performed the operation. The man approached for that purpoſe; when the lunatic ſuddenly ſtarting up, cut the throat of his keeper in ſuch a manner as nearly to ſever his head from his body.

This caſe preſents a ſtriking leſſon to thoſe to whoſe care lunatics are entruſted; and inſtructs them to be aware of credulity and miſtaken indulgence, as the ſubſequent does of the fatal neglect of confinement, when words and actions correſpond to manifeſt a depraved judgment, and a diſtempered imagination, in the unhappy caſe of Captain Hamilton, who recently ſhot himſelf in Abbey-Lane, Dublin, which was what might have been expected from his being permitted to go abroad unguarded when under the direful effects

effects of infanity. For three years he had been very confpicuous for extravagant expreffion, both in public and private life. During two feffions of parliament it was his cuftom to ftation himfelf in the gallery, and impede fome of the moft celebrated orators in their moft favourite fpeeches, with "*That's a lie.* The peo-" ple you reprefent know you to be a " fon of a b——, picking their pockets, " and ftealing their liberties," which behaviour feveral times occafioned fome alarm and confufion. This unfortunate gentleman was poffeffed of nearly £1000 per annum, and had loft an eye in the naval fervice. To make certain of his deftruction, he loaded two piftols, one he applied to the upper part of his mouth, and the other to his left ear. Having difcharged them both, his exit was immediately accomplifhed. It was cuftomary with the above extraordinary charafter, to enter many churches and chapels on the fabbath day, and pronounce on the fervice, that however the fubjeft might be good, it was a damned bad prafice. He was

dreffed

dreffed in a navy uniform, and making an allowance for his mental deprivation, he was efteemed a man of fpirit and politenefs.

Amongft the fatal effects of lunatics being too foon liberated from their confinement, the following will not be found the leaft horrible. About noon on the 23d of Auguft 1789, in Effex-Street, London, a fervant girl of Mr. Loader, who rented the parlour of a houfe, alarmed the neighbourhood by fcreaming out " For God's fake ! help ! a man is killing " my miftrefs." Two ticket porters immediately entered the houfe, and found Mrs. Loader with two dreadful ftabs in her neck, and Mr. Loader ftanding over her with a knife reeking with blood in his hand, whom they immediately fecured, but not before he had ftabbed himfelf three times in the lower part of his belly. The lady was taken to a furgeon in the fame ftreet. Mr. Loader had for fome time laboured under a ftate of infanity, and had been twice confined in a place properly appropriated for the reception

of

of perfons in his unfortunate fituation,
and from whence he had been recently
liberated on the fatal erroneous fuppofition of his being thoroughly reftored to
his reafon.   Mrs. Loader died two days
afterwards in confequence of her wounds,
and he furvived her but a few days longer.

At Poole, early in the morning of the
4th of Auguft 1793, a moft horrid murder was committed by a man on his wife,
and two children of about five and fix
years of age.   The circumftances of the
murder were nearly as follows.   The
man, who difcovered fymptoms of infanity, was confined in a place appropriate
for lunatics in the poor-houfe, where he
remained for fome time, and was at length
permitted to return home to his wife,
and continued for fome time quiet and
compofed, and feemed to be perfectly
reftored to his fenfes.   Having fome
wood to cleave, he borrowed a carpen-
ter's axe, and did it as well as any perfon
could in their proper fenfes.   In the evening he and his wife went to bed together,
as he intended going in a fhip that was to

fail

fail in the morning for America; but about four o'clock he arofe, and with the axe he had borrowed, perpetrated the horrid crime by cleaving all their fkulls; and what added to the dreadfulnefs of the murder, was the poor woman's being far gone in her pregnancy. He would like-wife have murdered a man that lodged in the houfe, had he not made his efcape, and given the alarm to the neighbours. The man's name was Jofeph Oakum; he was tried at the affizes at Poole, and found guilty of murder in a fit of infanity.

On the 21ft of May 1794, the infane fon of Lady Browne, of Brompton, ow-ing to the negligence of the perfon that had the care of him, efcaped from his own apartment, and furioufly rufhed into thofe of his mother, when feizing a poker, he inftantly murdered her by repeated blows on the head, and fled towards Buckingham-houfe; having fcaled the garden-walls of which, he was at length fecured in one of the plantations.

The murder of Sir Francis Kinlock, of Grimeftone, in Scotland, by his bro-ther,

ther, a lunatic, now Sir Archibald Kinlock, is so recent in the memory of the
public, as perhaps to render it unneceffary
to recite the horrid particulars. Let it
fuffice then to remark, that after he was
liberated from confinement, and was permitted to vifit his unfortunate brother,
upon being afked by his fervant whither
he was going, and when he fhould return,
he gave for anfwer, As foon as he had
killed his brother. No notice, however,
was taken of this fanguinary intention.
It was ftated on his trial before the high
court of jufticiary at Edinburgh, that
while in the Weft Indies he had been
feized with a fever, from which æra he
was never confidered to poffefs a found
mind, but was fubject to melancholy and
fits of jealoufy. At the time the unhappy deed was perpetrated, he was in
the moft lamentable ftate of derangement
of mind*.

C A S E

* Thefe and other horrid cataftrophes which have
happened from infanity, of which we have had fo
many recent inftances, particularly in the cafe of the
unhappy Mr, Medhurft, of Kippax, whofe trial for

Y   the

CASE LXXIV.

IT has been a generally received opinion, that perfons of the moft brilliant genius and lively imagination are moft fubject to madnefs; and that celebrated writer, Mr. Pope, feems to confirm the fuppofition in the following couplet:

> Great fenfe to madnefs is fo near allied,
> That thin partitions do the twain divide.

Infanity having been the immediate object of my practice for many years paft, I can fafely affirm that this obfervation is not generally founded in reality, and that madnefs proceeding from bodily complaints has no connection with the greater or leffer extent of the original powers of the foul, and may as frequently afflict the ignorant and the idiot, as the

the murder of his wife we have at length in the General Evening Poft of Tuefday the fifth of Auguft laft, fufficiently evince the neceffity of the timely removal of infane perfons to places of fecurity, thereby debarring them from the means and power of committing acts at which human nature fhudders.

philofopher

philofopher and the fcholar. When this terrible malady reduces a man of natural good fenfe and underftanding to the mental weaknefs of a child, its ravages on the human frame are more deplorable, and in a more intenfe degree wound the feelings of humanity. Endowed by nature with a brilliant fuperiority of mental powers, that were cultivated by a natural propenfity to learning, who did not lament the fate of poor Coleman, whofe diforder was not lefs methodical than fingular? From the wanderings of fuch a mind, if we cannot derive inftruction, we may at leaft obtain much ufeful humility. He ufed to fay, " That he died about two years fince, and was received with marks of uncommon favour into the courts of heaven; but that not perfectly liking his new fituation, he received permiffion to return to earth in whatever character he pleafed, and he accordingly affumed that of Prince of Shrewfbury." Reafoning rightly (as Locke, that great anatomift of the human mind, fays of perfons in his fituation) from

Y 2　　　　wrong

wrong premifes, he acted with fome cha-
racteriftic propriety, and in confequence
prefented his phyfician with an order for
£2000. Alas, poor human nature! He
died very lately, after having for many
years laboured under fuch a derangement
of his mental powers, that his friends
had no reafon to hope he would ever
emerge from the pitiable condition to
which he was reduced.

It has often been inconfiderately determined, that judgment may be eafily
formed on thofe cafes of mania that
require coercion. But decifions of this
nature cannot be eftablifhed but on the
cleareft and moft fatisfactory proof; and
when thus determined, great care and circumfpection are requifite at the period of
liberation, a period that can only be afcertained by thofe who have been accuftomed to be conftantly about them, as muft
be obvious to every perfon that has fuper-
intended the cure of maniacs; and vifi-
tants to houfes appropriated for the reception of fuch unhappy perfons, muft
have an uncommon fhare of acumen and
perfpicuity

perfpicuity to difcern the difference between thofe perfons that may be liberated
with fafety, and fuch whofe firft ufe of
liberty will be to deftroy themfelves or
others, or commit fome violent depreda-
tions on fociety. It requires a very nice
difcrimination to diftinguifh whether patients, who have apparently recovered
their fenfes, have been a fufficient time in
the *re-poffeffion of reafon*, to render it
fafe for them to return to their accuftomed
manner of life. For after recovery from
a ftate of infanity, the mind is during fome
period of time as weak as the body, after
violent difeafes. As in the latter inftance,
patients cannot immediately return to the
exercife and diet requifite in times of
health, without imminently endangering
a relapfe, fo in the former they cannot be
admitted to thofe objects that they were
accuftomed to behold before their mental
derangement, without hazarding an equal
or a greater danger. That perfons under
the influence of infanity are more *fubdo-
lous* than thofe afflicted with other indif-
pofitions, is an indifputable fact. And
the

the generality of maniacs poſſeſs ſuch a ſpecious plauſibility, as eaſily to deceive thoſe who are unaccuſtomed to their ſtratagems and deluſions; and it is very ſeldom, if ever, that they are found to act upon principles of veracity and gratitude. On the contrary, I can affirm from long experience that mendacity and ingratitude generally accompany them through every ſtage of this afflictive diſorder, often actuate them in their lucid intervals, until they are reſtored to a ſtate of convaleſcence; and as if a habitude was generated from madneſs, it ſeldom departs from them afterwards.

CASE LXXV.

I. T. an elderly man, who had been confined as a lunatic for ſome years, had ſufficient addreſs to impoſe upon thoſe who were legally appointed to inſpect the place of his reſidence. Through their interpoſing in their official capacity he obtain-

ed

ed his liberation, contrary to the wifhes
of his friend, and to thofe who were better acquainted with the ftate of his mind.
He had not obtained his liberty more than
four days, before he ftripped himfelf ftark
naked, and ran through the ftreets of a
neighbouring town, exclaiming that he
had been ftripped and plundered by a
banditti of robbers; that the keeper of
the houfe where he had been confined,
mentioning his name, owed him four mil-
lions of money, that he was firft coufin to
the Holy Ghoft, and many other abfurd
actions and expreffions, that made it neceffary to fecure him, fimilar to his former
reftrictions, in another houfe, where he remained feven years, and is but lately dead.
To this cafe might be added fome others,
delineative that hafty *official interference* is
equally prejudicial to the patient and practitioner; and which might prove a ufeful
memento to *delegated authority*, to cau-
tioufly and impartially inveftigate and ma-
turely deliberate on the cafe before they
attempt to decide on the propriety of
giving freedom to dementated individuals.

C A S E

CASE LXXVI.

A Gentleman of Mincing-Lane, London, who had been fome years a patient in my houfe, on a fudden became fo cool, collected, and rational, for a confiderable time, as to induce his relations to confent to his returning to his own houfe, where he received the congratulations of his friends, and for a few days conducted himfelf with every poffible degree of propriety; but early one morning he arofe haftily from his bed, threw up the fafh window of his apartment, and jumped from the elevation of three pair of ftairs into the ftreet. By the fall he fractured his fkull, and was otherwife fo much hurt, that he died in a few days afterwards.

CASE LXXVII.

A Gentleman, about forty years of age, by profeſſion a mathematical inſtrument-maker, and who became my patient in 1792, had been for ſeveral years in a ſtate of inſanity. During the continuance of ſome weeks he diſplayed ſigns of returning reaſon, and contrary to my opinion his friends concluded to give him a trial of liberty in a private family, before he was permitted to return home. This experiment was accordingly put in practice, and for ſome days he appeared perfectly cool, collected, and in his right ſenſes, and converſed in a uniform and rational manner; but not being at dinner on the ſixth day after his removal, he was ſought after, and his body was found in a pond about a mile diſtant from the houſe.

Many other circumſtances of a ſimilar nature might be adduced to demonſtrate the danger of too precipitately and implicitly confiding in the repreſentations and appearances of ſuch unfortunate perſons,

however

however fpecious or plaufible their arguments. There are amongft them fome
whofe converfation is highly proper
and rational, till fome particular topic
that lies dormant, and rankles in their
minds, becomes the fubject of converfation; then their infanity breaks forth into
action. Thus amidft the moft convin-
cing proofs of a well-cultivated under-
ing, enriched with knowledge, fuch as is
the greateft intellectual feaft for human
beings; touch but the favourite ftring,
however flightly, and the mental faculties
immediately lofe all their harmony, and
terminate in difcord and derangement.
An exemplification of this truth is evinced
in the following circumftance.

Some years fince, Mr. Burke vifited St.
Luke's, with an intention to inquire into
the general ftate of infanity in that hofpital; during this vifit he converfed with
a man for near an hour, on a variety of
topics, on which he expreffed himfelf with
fuch propriety and correctnefs, that Mr.
Burke expreffed his furprize to the keeper
that he was not difcharged. The keeper,
who

who well knew the particular species of
insanity under which he laboured, dictated
to him this interrogatory, " How he liked
his dinner?" which instantly caused him
to rave, and declare that it was poison,
from which nothing could divert his attention. Mr. Burke was now perfectly satis-
fied with the propriety of his confinement.

In the Commentaries of Van Swieten,
vol. 3d, aphorism 1094, p. 473, the author observes that he remembers to have
seen a man of sound mind in every respect,
who having heard that many persons had
been bitten with a mad dog, and had tried
the most approved methods, but were
seized with the hydrophobia, took the notion into his head that as the surgeon had
probably bled with the same lancets, in
bleeding other people, that dreadful poison might be spread and diffused through
a number of people in whom the disorder
had not yet made its appearance, and
might by them be communicated to
others; therefore to avoid this calamity,
he would not suffer a single mortal to
touch

touch him, and notwithstanding his good sense in other respects, not even his affection for his wife and children could make him deviate from this resolution.

I have had the care of a man upwards of eighteen years, who though tolerably well and rational in every other respect, can scarcely ever be persuaded to take his hand from his head, for fear that it should fall on his shoulders. Another, who although consistent in most other matters, always prefers walking in a retrograde manner; the reason for which he says is to prevent his meeting any person whom he dislikes, and to preserve his shoes from wearing out at the toes; and he is so irregular in walking the streets, as to induce those who observe him to point and laugh at him for a fool. Sometimes he is very deliberate in his gait, as if absorbed in meditation; at others quickening his step, accompanying it with ludicrous attitudes; but for the most part is fond of walking backward for the reasons before assigned.

Sauvages mentions the case of a physician,

fician, who after having been cured of a fever, imagined that he had been poifoned by the apothecary. Another, of a rich man, who imagined himfelf reduced to poverty, and who would not ftir out of bed for fear of wearing out his clothes, but in every other refpect was reafonable; and of a third, who believed himfelf a dunghill cock, and occupied himfelf in crowing and imitating the noife which that animal makes when it flaps its wings. I have alfo read of a man whofe legs were encircled with hay-bands, who upon being afked what was the nature of his complaint, affured the inquirer with a melancholy countenance that he beheld a general vitrification had begun to take place in his whole perfon, that his legs were converted into glafs bottles; that was it not for the protection afforded by the hay-bands, he fhould continually be in danger of breaking his own legs, and wounding his neighbours.

Cafper Borlæus, an orator, poet, and phyfician, who was not ignorant of the danger of fuch conduct, had fo injured the

the fenforium by too intenfe application to ftudy, that he believed his body was made of butter, and anxioufly avoided going near a fire, left he fhould melt away; till being weary of thofe apprehenfions, he put an end to his life by throwing himfelf into a well. And on the authority of Slochenetius, we hear of a man, who feared left Atlas, who is faid to fupport the world, fhould become weary of his exceffive load, and caft it off from him, and he and the reft of mankind fhould perifh in the general ruin. Reverius alfo relates the ftory of others, who would not make water left a deluge fhould be produced.

In the Med. Obferv. of Tulpius, lib. 1. cap. 18. we have an account of a painter of confiderable reputation in his art, who imagined that all his bones were become fo foft and pliant that they muft neceffarily bend like wax if he attempted to walk, or if any hard body was ftruck againft them. In conformity with the fears which fuch a notion infpired, he kept his bed during the whole winter,

imagining

imagining that if he arofe his legs would be compreffed with their own weight.

Marcus Donatus, in his Hift. Med. fpeaks of a baker at Ferrara, who believed he was made of butter, and on that account would not approach the oven left he fhould melt. And the fame author mentions a perfon of the name of Vicentinus, who believed he was of fuch an enormous fize that he could not go through the door of his apartment. His phyficians gave orders that he fhould forcibly be led through it, which was done accordingly, but not without a fatal effect, for Vicentinus cried out as he was forced along that the flefh was torn from his bones, and that his limbs were broken off, of which terrible impreffion he died in a few days, accufing thofe who conducted him with being his murderers.

I am favoured with the cafe of a female patient, now in Bedlam, which though not very interefting, may be allowed infertion for the many eccentric ideas fhe entertains. She is reprefented as one of thofe maniacs whofe conduct is uniformly correct,

correct, and who manages the ordinary concerns of life with great propriety, but whose head is filled with as much absurdity as ever entered the brain of any miserable being; that she is now about sixty years of age, and has been disordered in her intellects more than thirty years; that she has had three daughters, two of whom (the two eldest) have been insane, and one son, who lately died maniacal. For a considerable time together she did not betray any symptoms of insanity, her conversation was correct on ordinary topics, and her behaviour equally unexceptionable. She one day, however, expressed a wish to be liberated from her confinement, and upon being asked how she came into the hospital? she replied, it was an act of great injustice, and done with a view to deprive her of an immense property which she possessed, and she offered a douceur of £20,000 to any one who would release her from Bedlam, saying, her case was very hard, and wishing that when she died some years ago that she had never come to life again. On asking her

her how fhe came a fecond time into exiftence, fhe replied, that feveral years ago fhe
perfectly recollected lying in bed in a ftate
of extreme weaknefs, and being only able
to take nourifhment by teafpoons full, and
whilft her friends were feeding her, fhe
felt her foul depart from her body, and
heard her teeth clinch together on the
fpoon; that fhe then perceived her fpirit
gently and reluctantly flying off, gradually afcending upwards, having two cir-
cumferences of glory round her; that her
body was then conveyed to the chancel
of the church, where it remained fome
weeks, when fuddenly a tall dark-com-
plexioned man, with his hair curled all
over, fpoke to her; he was the Almighty;
and fhe inftantly became alive, and was
imperceptibly conveyed to her own
home: when arrived at the door, fhe faw
her fon, but he had no hair on his head;
inftead of hair it was covered with icicles
of white fugar-candy, and ftudded with
carraway comfits. This woman alfo fup-
pofes herfelf to be poffeffed of a certain
power over a fet of beings, whom fhe

z   terms

terms the Congo Devils, and often retires
of an afternoon to her cell to maintain
fome very fharp conflicts with thofe diabolical adverfaries; and on many occafions declares fhe is obliged to hurl ninety
tons of cannon balls at them, and having a
powerful and unerring hand, the flaughter
on fome occafions is immenfe. She does
not, however, pretend to deny that in one
inftance fhe came off but fecond beft, one
of the chiefs of the Congo men, with un-
paralleled impudence, and dreffed like
one of the lord-mayor's footmen, fhe fays,
made a ferious attack on her chaftity, but
how far he prevailed is a fecret, and fuch
will ever remain. On inquiry who thefe
Congo Devils were, fhe faid, that when
Satan was on his travels he vifited Africa,
and refided a long time in the kingdom of
Congo, where debauching the wives and
daughters of the good people of that
country, he created a numerous offspring,
who through holes, crannies, and bye-
places, foon worked their way into Europe.

Amongft the number of fudden recoveries

from

from infanity, the following cafe deferves to be recorded. A poor itinerant lunatic woman, near Stone, in Bedfordfhire, threw herfelf into a well, near twenty feet deep, in the bottom of which was about five feet of water; fhe no fooner found her fituation painful and inconvenient, than fhe began to cry out for help, when a ladder being put down, fhe afcended it of her own accord, to the aftonifhment of all the beholders, without having received the leaft injury. What made this the more extraordinary was, that fhe inftantly recovered her mental faculties.

Daniel Millfham, a poor labouring man, in the parifh of Dilciam, in Norfolk, who had been deprived of his fenfes more than twenty years, and for the laft twelve years chained down to the floor of a chamber in a fmall cottage in the village, attended by his mother, and maintained by his brother, was one day found ftretched out on the floor, apparently dead. On the return of her fon from his work, fhe told him that Daniel was dead, when he went to the chamber, and finding his brother

ftill

ſtill warm, and calling him by his name, Daniel inſtantly roſe, and aſked him what he wanted, and from that moment reco-vered his perfeƈt ſenſes. He had not had any cloaths on for more than ten years. His beard, that had grown to an amazing length, was cut off, and he has been ever ſince rational and regular in his conduƈt, and in a few days was entirely recovered.

During the extraordinary inundation that happened at Glaſgow in 1791, the water ran ſo high as to reach the cells of the mad-houſe. The dread of the water had an inſtantaneous and wonderful effeƈt upon the lunatics, rendering the whole of them, even the moſt furious, quiet and traƈtable. They trembled like children, and ſuffered themſelves to be conduƈted to apartments in the upper ſtory, where they remained calm and peaceable as long as the court-yard continued covered with water; but this effeƈt remained no longer than while the objeƈt of terror was in view.

Van Helmont tells us of a certain car-penter of Antwerp, who fancied he had
ſeen

feen fome frightful fpeétres in the night, that he entirely loft his fenfes; he was therefore fent to the tomb of the Holy Virgin St. Dympofa, whom they profefs to cure thofe who are poffeffed of evil fpirits. The patient was boarded there for nearly a whole year, and though evidently a madman, the ufual means were employed, but no money being remitted from Antwerp, for the laft fix months, he was fent home bound in a carriage. Having found means to extricate himfelf on his journey, he leaped from the carriage, and threw himfelf into a deep pool which was near, from which after fome time he was taken out, apparently dead, and replaced in the carriage; he recovered, however, in confequence of this fudden immerfion, and lived eight years afterwards entirely free from mania.

CASE

CASE LXXVIII.

MR. P——, an eminent attorney in this county, who had laboured under mental derangement for more than twenty years, without receiving the leaft relief from the advice and affiftance of myfelf and many other medical practitioners, was on a fudden reftored to the natural plenitude of his intellectual faculties on hearing the news of his fon's death, and from that period continued to tranfact the bufinefs of his profeffion with uninterrupted correctnefs and propriety for more than two years, never difcovering the leaft trait of his former malady; till one morning, when not coming down ftairs at his ufual time, he was difcovered in bed to have divided the arteries in both wrifts with a penknife, the confequent effufion of blood from which had reduced him to fo low and weak a ftate, that although he made many attempts to fpeak, he could not be underftood, was totally unable to fwallow any

kind

kind of fuſtenance, and after languiſhing
a few hours, expired.

Inſtances of recovery from mania, by
the patient being ſuddenly immerſed in
cold water, have been ſo numerous, as to
have induced the experiment of cold
bathing, the application of the clay cap,
ice, and bonnet of ſnow; and ſome inſtances of cure have certainly occurred
from the uſe of the ſhower bath, which
by its ſudden effect poured unawares upon the patient, deſerves the preference in
my opinion to any other immerſion, when
advantage is expected from that mode of
treatment; but in general the unmanage-
able ſtate of the patients when furiouſly
infane, and to whom theſe applications
are uſually made, often prevents the effects of ſuch remedies towards a cure. I
never ſaw but one infane patient that
could be ſaid to be cured by cold bathing;
but in the melancholy temperament, with
great tenſion of the fibres, have often
known abundant ſervice derived from
the warm bath.

CASE

CASE LXXIX.

A Gentleman of fortune in this county, who had long habituated himfelf to a courfe of intemperance, was in June 1792, fuddenly afflicted with the internal piles, which occafioned great pain and uneafinefs upon the voiding of his excrements. He had fpoken lightly of the complaint, but had never taken any thing to mitigate its violence; his ideas became confufed, and he fupected that poifon was infufed into every thing that was offered to him, a fufpicion moft commonly attached to confirmed mania. He laboured under much anxiety and fear, was alternately loud and turbulent, fullen, and inclined to mifchief. Coercion became neceffary, and my advice was folicited; he complained of a fevere head-ache, his eye-lids looked fore, and were tumefied almoft to fuppuration; he loft his recollection, had fpafms of the mufcles of the face, with involuntary action of the fingers and biting

of

of the nails; his pulfe was ftrong, full, hard, and frequent; his belly was tenfe, fore, and fub-elaftic; his eyes were in continual motion. He immediately loft twelve ounces of blood, that had a yellow cruft on its furface; was ordered to take the foluble tartar every other day in barley-water, and at intervals a camphorated mixture. He was bled again on the third day, and by pe...evering in a proper courfe of medicine, and a cooling regular diet, he foon recovered intirely from mental derangement, as well as its primary caufe, the piles.

CASE LXXX.

A Gentleman of an atrabilarious temperament and fedentary life, and who derived hypochondriafm from his anceftors, had for fome time been afflicted with hæmorrhoidal tumours at the lower part of the inteftinum rectum; they had bled co-

pioufly,

pioufly, but ceafing all at once he became
furioufly agitated with confufed ideas,
fubject to violent paffions, his eye-lids
were in conftant vibration, he devoured
his aliment with voracioufnefs, and when
I firft faw him on the 24th of September
1791, he had not been at ftool for four
days. The pulfe juftifying the operation,
fix ounces of blood were taken from his
arm, which was very buffy. Cooling aperients and regimen were prefcribed, the
warm pediluvium was ufed at bed-time,
and bleeding repeated, and in a few days
the patient was intirely reftored to health.

I have been informed by a gentleman
eminent for his knowledge of maniacal
complaints, that in two different inftances
of fuppreffion of the hæmorrhoids, the
moft permanent affiftance was rendered to
the patient by the exhibition of acrid
purgatives of the aloetic kind.

The fudden death of the late Mr.
Dawes, of the Univerfity of Cambridge,
having furprized his family and acquaintance, he having been a man of cheerful
temper

temper and in good circumſtances, it has
ſince been diſcovered that he was very
much afflicted with the piles, and which
during the paroxyſm have been frequently
obſerved to produce a temporary inſanity,
as in the preſent inſtance.

CASE LXXXI.

INSANE perſons too often loſe that
natural delicacy and cleanlineſs which it is
the incumbent duty of all human beings
to preſerve to the utmoſt of their power.
What can be a greater degradation of the
human character, than when the conſtitution is diſpoſed to feed vermin? I cannot
inſert it as a fact within my own knowledge, but I have every reaſon to believe
the truth of the relation, of a maniac in
the neighbourhood of Hoxton, who was
literally deſtroyed by the ſwarms of pediculi that infeſted and covered all parts
of his body. I well knew a young gentleman

tleman of a pituitous habit, who in the
year 1789, was attacked with a melancholy fpecies of infanity, and in a dark
moment of defpair attempted to put an
end to his exiftence, which to ufe his own
expreffion was become *infupportable;* it
was therefore neceffary to adopt the utmoft
vigilance for the future prefervation of his
perfon ; and it is no lefs fingular than
true, that when he enjoyed a lucid interval a few days, he was always attacked
with the morbus pediculofus, that difappeared when he reverted into a deranged
ftate of mind, and as conftantly recurred when he had a lucid interval, for
the fpace of four years, during which
time he was in confinement ; from which
however he was removed under the idea
of his being in a better ftate of mind than
he really was, as I find upon inquiry the
return of his mental derangement made
the fame meafure again neceffary, and
that he continues to be more than ever infefted with his pediculous complaint.

CASE

CASE LXXXII.

AN elderly lady, of the Ifle of Thanet, that was infane, whofe fkin was always thick, rough, and greafy, owing to an elephantiafis, for which fhe had gone through feveral courfes of alterative medicines, alternately confifting of antimonials and mercurials, was fo much difpofed to pediculi in her head and body, that notwithftanding every attention to cleanlinefs, and the repeated ufe of powder of quick-lime, mercurial lotions, and liniments, (which ferved but as palliatives) it was impoffible to keep her free from them for any length of time together. When fhe was removed by her friends from motives of œconomy, this difagreeable affection was imputed to neglect in thofe who had attended her, till the experience of her relations convinced them of the injuftice of the cenfure, and that the imputation was intirely unfounded.

CASE

CASE LXXXIII.

A YOUNG lady of fingular worth and amiablenefs, who had been advifed to have an iffue in her arm for a fcorbutic affection at the age of twelve years, when arrived at the age of maturity, being engaged in a matrimonial contraɛt, fhe without confulting any perfon, fuffered the iffue to dry up, which produced in her fuch maniacal fymptoms, as induced her friends to apply for my advice. I faw her on the 12th of April 1794, and upon inquiry found that the iffue had been healed about fix weeks, and that in a few days afterwards fhe became dull, gloomy, and dejeɛted; complained of a fevere head-ache, with fugitive palenefs, impaired hearing, yawning, and ftretching, inflamed eye-lids, want of appetite, inceffant change of pofture, and had a peculiar wildnefs in her looks; her ideas were perpetually varying from one objeɛt to another. I prefcribed an antimonial emetic, and direɛted a feton to be paffed be-

tween

tween the fhoulders in the direction of the fpine, and three times a day naufeating dofes of antim. tart. to be given. In a few days the feton difcharged plentifully, and in lefs than a fortnight every fymptom of mania difappeared. Laxatives were recommended, and tonics occafionally given. The feton being fore and painful, was now dried up, and the iffue being opened in the fame fituation as before, the patient has continued well ever fince.

C A S E   LXXXIV.

A YOUNG man of refpectable family in the county of Suffex, who had for fome days felt confiderable pain and uneafinefs from an eryfipelatous eruption on his face, neck, and back part of his head, was advifed to foment thofe parts with forge-water, in which fome vitriolated zinc had been diffolved. This occafioned a tranflation of the humour to the brain, and

and drove him raving mad. In this ſtate,
November 1794, he became my patient;
was bled *ad deliquium*, had a ſeton *inter ſcapulas* in the direction of the ſpine,
and by following the antiphlogiſtic plan
both of diet and medicine, he obtained a
complete cure.

CASE LXXXV.

IN two caſes where maniacal patients
experienced a partial recovery from having
contracted the itch, ſo in this particular inſtance mania appears to have been brought
on in conſequence of a retroceſſion of that
diſorder.   The patient was a ſtrong, luſty,
middle-aged man, whoſe children had for
ſome time been troubled with the itch,
but were now in a ſtate of recovery; he
had hitherto eſcaped infection, but at
length the complaint appeared on his
hands, between his fingers, round his
waiſt, and in his arm-pits; he had recourſe for a cure to an advertiſed noſtrum,
which

which upon the fecond application repelled the eruption, and he was in confequence foon after attacked with mania
furibunda. In this ftate I found him; his
pulfe was full, hard, and tenfe; his refpiration difficult; his face and eyes tumid
and inflamed, and the febrile impetus exceffive. I directed venefection *ad deliquium,* a veficatory between the fhoulders,
and in the evening an antimonial emetic,
which not operating as was expected, produced a ftool. An emollient clyfter was
given with due effect. His regimen was
chiefly barley-water, panada, and whey;
every fix hours he took a faline draught,
with vin. antimoniale and camphorated
julep. On the third day of my attendance I found the patient calm and reafonable; he had perfpired freely, and his
pulfe was reduced nearly to its natural
ftandard; but as he ftill complained of a
pain in his head and ftomach, I ordered
another emetic and a repetition of the
bleeding, which gave him immediate relief. The emetic, as in the firft inftance, operated only by ftool, but in a

A a few

few days his recovery was completed. As there are fometimes eruptions fimilar to the itch, which prove contagious, it is not improbable that this might have been of that defcription, and by a fudden repulfion to the brain, have occafioned fuch violent excitement as to prove the caufe of this delirium.

CASES LXXXVI. and LXXXVII.

DURING the lucid intervals in confirmed cafes of mania, there is generally to be obferved fome certain prognoftics of its return. A young woman of cacheftic habit, who had been infane from her fifteenth year, had always a lucid interval during her menftruation, at the termination of which fhe reverted to her ufual ftate of mental derangement, and continued fo till the return of the flux, which was very regular, but in fmall quantity, and fhe was then again clear and rational.

A lady

A lady who had every fpring and fall been afflicted with periodical madnefs, was for feveral days previous to its return obferved to be more than ordinarily pale and fallow, with a florid countenance and heat of the head; and to have a peculiar look with her eyes, unufual at other times.

A gentleman who had been many years under my care, and who for fome months together did not difcover the leaft traits of a difordered imagination, always became furious and infane in a few days after a flight tumefaction and rednefs appeared on the ciliary glands, attended with fugitive palenefs.

C A S E LXXXVIII.

THE wife of A. M. a middle-aged woman of a delicate conftitution, after labouring under a train of nervous and hyfterical affections for more than twelve months, became intirely infane, and by repeated bleedings was fo much debilitated with extenuation of the whole body, as to prefent a fpectacle of mifery and horror. In this evidently reduced ftate of

the

the folids, I had recourfe to a proper diet and medicines beft adapted to the cure of a relaxed ftate of the folids, preceded by a gentle antimonial emetic; bark and opium in fmall quantities were given at proper intervals, and continued for fome weeks, when fhe had confiderably recruited her ftrength, and evinced evident figns of returning reafon, and by a farther perfeverance in thefe remedies, fhe entirely recovered her fenfes. It was remarkable that before her derangement fhe had always retained an antipathy to opium, but fhe has fince fhewed fuch a fondnefs for the ufe of that remedy as to determine her never to be without it, and on the leaft fymptom of her former complaint, fhe has immediate recourfe to its affiftance.

CASES LXXXIX. XC. and XCI.

THAT great and fudden emotions proceeding from fear and terror are frequently productive of an aberration of thought and reafon, is fully exemplified in the three

fucceding

fucceeding cafes, each of which came under my own knowledge.

In the year 1784, Mr. W. a young gentleman of genteel and refpectable connexions, was placed very early in life at a public feminary, where he was fo much terrified by being locked into a dark room by one of his fchool-fellows, out of a mere frolic, as to lofe his reafon, and he has never fince emerged from a ftate of the moft deplorable idiotifm.

I. T. the fon of a merchant in London, about the thirteenth year of his age, was fo terrified by the appearance of a man difguifed in a white fheet, for the purpofe of frightening his fellow-fervants, as to fall into a ftrong convulfive fit. After his life had been for many days defpaired of, he recovered, but never had the proper ufe of his fpeech; he articulated his words very incoherently, and became quite an idiot; was afflicted with epileptic fits, and died of them in the fixteenth year of his age.

The fon of a counfellor of great celebrity

lebrity in his profeſſion, was from a
fright, from being a boy of the moſt hope-
ful and promiſing intellects, reduced to
the mental weakneſs of an idiot, and to
this hour continues in that unfortunate
ſituation, retaining in his aſpect a mixture
of that terror the object firſt excited.
Van Swieten relates a remarkable caſe
of a woman, who was frightened in the
night by a ſudden alarm of thieves attempting to enter through her chamber-
window; and whenever ſhe was drop-
ping to ſleep, would awake in a fright, although ſhe knew that the ſervants ſat up
to guard the houſe every night. This
terror was never overcome, and was par-
ticulary prevalent towards the evening,
when ſhe always began to tremble, grow
pale, and look as if ſhe ſuſpected ſome
evil deſign upon her perſon. Her anxiety
in a ſhort time terminated in an uncon-
querable melancholy.

In the corporal effects of fear we have
many well-atteſted caſes of the hair of the
head having ſuddenly changed grey; and
frequent

frequent inftances of its having produced epilepfy and convulfions, are recorded by authors of indubitable veracity: and amongft thofe complicated with infanity and melancholy, we find the following cafes in Greeding's Effays on the Ufe and Virtue of the Veratrum Album. " J. C. V. " a young man, twenty-three years of age, " was in his eighth year fuddenly fright- " ened by a dog, the impreffion of which " frequently occurred to him in the night; " being then always tormented with the " idea of being attacked by the animal, " he was taken with epilepfy, which " recurred every half year, but which af- " ter fome time returned every month; " he was alfo afflicted with borborygmi, " want of appetite, and violent head-ache " which difturbed his reft. Weaknefs of " underftanding and real delirium enfued, " and continued feveral days together, " which fymptoms after a continuance of " three weeks were fucceeded by vertigo. " J. C. B. a miner, aged thirty-four, of fhort " ftature, and being of a mufcular, flefhy

" make,

" make, was brought into our workhoufe
" on the fifth of February 1770, on ac-
" count of an obftinate melancholy which
" had commenced in the autumn of 1769,
" in confequence of terror from an ima-
" ginary caufe, of which when he was
" afked concerning it he gave the follow-
" ing account, That he had always enjoyed
" good health till laft fummer, but on one
" day during that feafon as he was enter-
" ing the fmelting-houfe alone, a horrid
" big black human figure fuddenly jump-
" ed on his fhoulders, and terrified him fo
" as to occafion his prefent diforder."

In feveral cafes of maniacal affections, attended with hyfterical or convulfive fpafms,
I have adminiftered mufk with fome degree of fuccefs; I fay with fome degree,
becaufe in very few inftances could the
cure be afcribed to the ufe of that article
alone.   Its adminiftration has ever appeared to me moft efficacious, when joined with camphor, and moft to be depended
on when taken in the form of pills; but
in general the circumftances of the patient,

tient, the high price of the drug, and the difficulty of procuring it genuine, have proved objections to that extenfive ufe of it which might have teftified the celebrity which fome authors have afcribed to it, confidering it as one of the moft powerful antifpafmodics in the whole materia medica.

The late ingenious Dr. Wall, in his Medical Tracts, has favoured us with the following accounts, that from the extraordinary fingularity of the relation, are well deferving a place in this publication. He obferves, that from the efficacy of mufk, in curing delirium, he conceived it would be of ufe in curing maniacal diforders. " I happened," continued he, " about a year and a half ago, to fay fo in the prefence of a gentleman at Oxford, whofe fon had been for fome time exceedingly difordered in his fenfes by a difappointment in love; being unable to fleep, refufing fuftenance, and attempting to throw himfelf out of the window of a high room where he was confined. The father begged of me to give him the medicine, and affured me that he would make ufe of it,

as

as the methods previously adopted had proved ineffectual. He soon returned me a letter of thanks, acquainting me that the medicine had made his son sleep foundly for twenty-four hours, and that he had perspired plentifully, and waked in his proper senses ; and has since heard that from being a mere skeleton, he has grown remarkably corpulent."

In the next case he observes that a particular friend of his went mad about a year and a half before, when he mentioned the preceding case to two gentlemen who attended the patient, and with their approbation gave him musk, native and factitious cinnabar, of each a scruple in a gill of arrack. In about three hours he fell asleep, which supposing to be the effect of the medicine, they left him, and soon after they were gone he awoke, but the next day not appearing any better, he was removed to a proper place of confinement. Nothing else was prescribed for him, but at night he slept foundly, appeared much better the next day, and continued mending until he became intirely well. How much

much of the cure might be attributed to
the effects of this medicine, he does not
take upon him to affert, as it did not operate immediately, nor in the ufual manner; but he mentions this, principally to
fhew that twenty grains of mufk at a dofe
had no ill effect, if it did not produce a
good one.

CASE XCII.

IN May 1793, I was confulted in the
cafe of a patient in the neighbourhood of
C——.   She was a young lady of the
moft polite and elegant manners, and diftinguifhed for the moft amiable mildnefs
and complacency of temper.   She had
been in a ftate of nervous languor and
dejection of fpirits for feveral weeks; fhe
became melancholy, fhewed a great averfion to fociety, and a predominant love of
folitude; every object alarmed her mind,
every paffion was tremblingly alive, and
every place defart and forlorn; her heart

was

was fhut againft every pleafing fenfation,
and her mind difmiffed every chearing
fentiment; at intervals fhe was troubled
with the globus hyftericus, with general
fpafms, and almoft inceffantly with fpafmodic panting; fhe was averfe to food,
and took the fmalleft portion with reluctance. She received me with much compofure, and defcribed her cafe with elo-
quence and fenfibility. " Her habitation,"
fhe faid, " was no longer comfortable, no
longer the feat of health, or the refidence
of calm repofe; but her foul was loft, and
fhe defpaired of happinefs in a future
ftate." Her intellect appeared faftened
upon this dreadful idea. Upon inquiry I
found that infanity had never fhewn itfelf
in any branch of her pedigree, and that
her mind had been perplexed and infatuated by the infinuations of a female acquaintance, who had ftrongly imbibed the
taint of religious enthufiafm, and had frequently talked to her in the moft frantic
ftrains of vifions, prophecies, loft mercy,
and the torments of a future ftate. This
obvioufly appeared to be the fource of
her

her delufion—her corporeal complaints approached to the hyfteric type. She had been fubject to an eruption of the herpetic kind about her breafts, fides, and the pit of her ftomach. Her tongue was foul, her pulfe quick and weak, her fkin pale and dry, and her eyes conftantly moving. She had perfpired but little, and her nights had been paffed without fleep. After recommending a change of refidence, prohibiting all intercourfe with her *religious* friend, giving directions refpecting her diet, and appointing a proper attendant to be always about her, I ordered an antimonial emetic to clear her ftomach, after which I prefcribed as follows:

R Mofch. orient optim. ʒijfs.
    Mucilag. Gum. Arab. q. s.
    Dividend in pilul. xx. capiat ij ter, quaterve in die.

with a draught of camphorated mixture after each dofe, and to be repeated in the night, in cafe of her being very reftlefs, with the addition of the fourth part of a grain of opium to the pills then given; the warm pediluvium was advifed at bed-time, and a feton a feton ordered to be paffed *inter fcapulas,* in the direction of the fpine.

After this procefs had been continued a few days, fhe became much more calm and compofed, with every appearance of convalefcence. At this crifis a truly pious divine of her acquaintance had free accefs to her, and fucceeded in endeavouring to enlighten the dark gloom that had involved her mind, and brought it back to a clear fenfe of religious duties ; and after the patient had continued completely rational for fix weeks, the feton was dried up, and fhe became in every refpect as well as at any period before her illnefs. The eruption did not appear for fome months after the cure, and then in a much lefs degree than ufual.

In the celebrated Dr. Zimmerman's fecond vol. of Solitude, page 192, we find an inftance fomewhat fimilar to the preceding hiftory. He fays that "in the courfe of his practice as a phyfician he was called upon to attend a young lady whofe natural difpofition had been extremely cheerful, until a fevere fit of ficknefs

nefs damped her fpirits, and rendered her averfe to all thofe lively pleafures which fafcinate the youthful mind. The debility of her frame, and the change of her temper, were not fufficiently attended to in the early ftages of her convalefcence; the anxiety of her mind was vifible in the altered features of her face, and fhe was frequently heard to exprefs a melancholy regret that fhe had confumed fo many hours in the frivolous though innocent amufements of the age. Time increafed by almoft imperceptible degrees thefe fymptoms of approaching melancholy; and they at length exhibited themfelves in penitential lamentations of the fin fhe had committed with refpect to the moft trifling actions of her life, and in which no fhadow of offence could poffibly be found. At the time he was called in, this fuperftitious melancholy was attended with certain indications of mental derangement. The diftemper clearly originated in the indifpofition of the body, and the gloomy apprehenfions which difeafe and pain had introduced into the mind during a period of many

3   months.

months. This once lively, handfome, but now almoft infane female, was daily attacked with fuch violent paroxyfms of her complaint, that fhe loft all fenfe of her fituation, and exclaimed in horrid diftraction and deep defpair, that her perdition was already come, and that the fiends were waiting to receive her foul, and plunge it into *the bittereft torments of hell*. Her conftitution, however, ftill fortunately retained fufficient ftrength to enable him by *the power of medicine* gradually to change its temperament, and to reduce that violence which had long been preying on her life; her mind became more even, in proportion as her nerves recovered their former tone; and when her intellectual powers were in a condition to be acted upon with effect, he fuccefsfully counteracted the baleful effects of *fuperftition* by the wholefome infufion of *real religion,* and reftored by degrees a lively, young, and virtuous woman. to her family and herfelf.

CASE

C A S E   XCIII.

A GENTLEMAN in a military capacity, who had been under an ill-managed courſe of mercurials, became inſane in 1794, and was placed under my care. His deglutition ſeemed painful and difficult; he was ſubject to frequent eructations; his eyes were continually moving with a vibration of the eye-lids; inceſſant change of poſture, great anxiety, and frequent delirium. He had no fever; his pulſe was hard and ſtrong; his ſkin ſqualid, hot, and dry; he ſlept but little; was inclined to be coſtive; ſpat about him in an indiſcriminate manner; often complained of coldneſs in his legs and thighs; ſighed much; thought every object was on fire; and was continually rubbing his head with his hands dipped in water, or any other liquid that was within his reach. He had been under a diſcipline that had apparently aggravated the diſorder, and made him worſe; a ſyſtem of mildneſs was adopted in its ſtead, friction to his legs

B b   and

and thighs, and the warm pediluvium,
were ufed every night and morning; ten
ounces of blood was taken from his arm,
and every other evening he took the following bolus:

R Sal Sodæ ʒſs.
  Calomel gr. i.
  Opii   gr. ½
  Syr. Zinzib. q. ſ. ut f. bolus.

Under this courſe, with occaſional laxatives,
he continued for the ſpace of three weeks,
when he appeared in every reſpect much
altered for the better, and expreſſed himſelf
gratefully ſenſible of the reverſe of treatment, and the indulgent attention that he
had experienced, and wiſhing to diſcontinue
his medicines, his requeſt was complied
with for a few days; but not continuing ſo
well as he was before, he was again bled,
took an emetic, and the alterative bolus
was repeated, with a decoction of ſarſapa-
rilla, ſome ſymptoms of a peculiar nature
inclining me to believe it neceſſary.   But
there ſtill remained great alienation of
mind, till an eruption of the herpetic kind
appearing on his ſtomach, back, and arms,
                              together

together with a general yellownefs of
the fkin, and particularly in the albugine-
ous coats of his eyes, this delivered him
from all mental perturbation; and the
fymptoms that had fupervened being removed by bleeding, and an attenuating
diet, he was perfectly re-eftablifhed in his
reafon. But a fecond time relapfing from
a fimilar caufe into the fame ftate as before, he was again committed to my care,
in Auguft 1795; when by a proper alterative courfe and regimen, very little
different from what had been ufed before,
after a few weeks, upon the appearance
of the fame cutaneous eruption, the event
proved falutary, and he left my houfe
entirely recovered.

CASE XCIV.

IT is a well-known and eftablifhed fact,
that intenfity of thought, and long protracted application of the mind to one
object, are common caufes of infanity.

A gen-

A gentleman of an atrabilarious temperament, ſtudiouſly diſpoſed, and naturally
ſubject to hypochondriaſis, by directing
his attention without interruption to phi-
loſophical ſubjects and experiments, became low-ſpirited, fretful, jealous, anxious,
and deſpondent; he complained of the
head-ache; his eye-lids were ſore and
ſuppurated; he had a nauſea, and frequent febrile redneſs, impaired viſion,
tawny ſpots on the ſkin, with a ſenſe of gid-
dineſs and fulneſs. It was obſerved that he
always expreſſed the utmoſt abhorrence
and indignation at any thing of a red colour. The curtain of the room, and a
waiſtcoat of that colour, he tore into a
thouſand pieces. He was coſtive, could
obtain no ſleep, often refuſed his ſuſte-
nance, and was much emaciated. He was
in this preciſe ſtate in April 1795. His
diſorder appeared confirmed, notwithſtanding a courſe of emetics, camphor,
muſk, the fœtid gums, the cold bath,
and a ſeton between the ſhoulders, had
ſeverally been made uſe of, excluſion
of diſagreeable *colours*, diminution of
light,

light, and the moſt gentle coercion. I was
not able to remove his diſorder; and in
three months after his admiſſion to my
houſe, he died of a hectic fever.

For ſeveral remarkably ſingular caſes
of infanity, from intenſe ſtudy, the reader
is referred to the works of the celebrated
Tiſſot. In this caſe the indignation excited
by particular colours ı. not more ſingular,
than the terror, fear, and averſion, that
other maniacs expreſs at particular objects.   I have at this time two female
patients of long ſtanding, who have both
ſuch a rooted enmity to cats, that whenever they can ſeize them they will tear
them to pieces with their hands, nails, or
teeth ; or will bite them through in ſome
part or other; ſo that the poor animals
coming in their way, ſeldom eſcape, at leaſt
without having their limbs broken or diſ-
located.

A gentleman who was placed under
my care for madneſs, accompanied with
epileptic fits, would at any time if he ſaw
a large fly, or waſp, have a fit; or even if
he heard the buzzing of their wings; and
was ſo much terrified if he ſaw a child
enter

enter the door, that he would immediately
fecrete himfelf by creeping under his bed,
or getting under the table.   Having once
efpied from his chamber window a child
playing in the ftreet, he ran down ftairs,
and actually got into and hid himfelf in
an oven to avoid the imaginary danger.

In maniacal cafes, combined with afci-
tes and anafarca, I have found the *digitalis*
of effential fervice.   And in one cafe of
melancholy, the patient being of a leuco-
phegmatic habit, attended with dyfpnœa,
fcarcity of urine, difturbed fleep, anafarcous
fwellings, and great alienation of mind, to
the repeated dofes of this excellent medicine, and the occafional application of
crem. tart. this patient entirely owed her
recovery, after many other remedies had
been tried in vain.   In one cafe of *mania
furibunda,* where the abdomen was greatly diftended with water, attended with a
perceptible fluctuation from percuffion,
it had been given from one grain to four
or five in a day, which by increafing
the flow of urine, reduced the abdomen
gradually, and with the affiftance of exercife

cife and a tonic regimen, this patient received an intire cure both in body and
mind. In maniacal affeations the corporeal part of the fyftem is fometimes violently affeaed, and fometimes not at all;
and fo feldom are maniacs the fubjeas of
dropfy, that in thirty years praatice I
never knew one inftance of it, except in
the cafes before recited.

CASE XCV.

IN confequence of long-continued vexation from a feries of misfortune, a young
man, refpeatably allied, of ftrong hereditary
predifpofition to mania, in the county of
Suffolk, became furioufly infane, and for
fome weeks was treated with the moft
rigorous coercion that could be adminiftered. The fpouting pot had been frequently ufed both for his food and medicine; a praatice in itfelf fo painfully unpleafant, that it ought never to be adopted
if it can poffibly be avoided, as it feldom
                              produces

produces any good effect. In November 1791, he was placed under my care, when he was furiously agitated with confused ideas, and appeared greatly emaciated; he had a peculiar wildnefs of his eyes, and fufpected poifon had been infufed into every thing that was offered to him; his pulfe was very full and hard, and he was fubject to eructations; his afpect was flufhed and inflated; eight ounces of blood were taken from his arm, that appeared black and grumous; antimonial emetics were repeatedly adminiftered; a feton was paffed between the fhoulders in the direction of the fpine, and a much milder treatment than before was adopted. At bed-time the camphorated mixture with opium was given with good effect. He became calm in the day, had quiet nights, and gradually recovered his health and reafon. He was difmiffed from my houfe at the end of eight months, and has continued well ever fince.

The gentle treatment in this cafe contributed much to his cure, and fhould always be adopted in preference to rigorous meafures,

meafures, where the cafes will admit of it. I likewife have the fatisfaction to add, that management and proper government under fuch unfortunate circumftances is often more to be depended on than medicine; but when both are judicioufly and humanely blended, the patient has always the beft chance of recovery.

Having fpoken againft the practice of *fpouting*, I fhall only add, that in two inftances of long-continued obftinate refufal of aliment, where the conftant ufe of the pot was advifed, by which fome liquid food was forced into the ftomach, the reftraint and violence attending the procefs increafed the maniacal fymptoms, and notwithftanding this and every other method that could be devifed, they were fo tenacious in their rejection of food, that after fome weeks both the patients died of mere inanition *.

CASE

* In fome cafes of obftinate abftinence, where the lives of the patients have been in imminent danger from *famine*, I have been well informed by a practitioner, whofe peculiar province affords him frequent opportunities of feeing patients in all the different ftages of mania, that he has found nothing fucceed better than ftrong *draftic*

purges

C A S E   XCVI.

JOHN SOMERS, a gilder by profes-
sion, was in June 1792 suddenly seized
with the dry colic, that was succeeded by
a paralytic affection of the left leg and
arm, and an incurvation of the fingers. An
inability to extend them succeeded, and a
dreadful train of symptoms that resisted
every method of relief, which being followed by mental derangement, induced
his friends to apply to me for advice. His
complexion was palid and sallow, he was
obstinately costive, had little appetite, was
subject to nausea, the cramp in his legs and
feet, and was frequently afflicted with contraction, pain, tension, and uneasiness about
the navel. Common purgatives had failed
of effect; recourse, therefore, was had to
others of a stronger nature, with more success; his respiration was difficult; and some
remains of a venereal affection evincing
that his disorder was not wholly attributable

purges repeated at proper intervals, and that in some
instances of this kind he has even given half an ounce
of jalap at a dose, with the best effect.

to

to his bufinefs, I commenced the cure with
an emetic, and afterwards gave him half a
grain of calomel every night and morning, the effects of which were vifible after the fifth day. Electricity was now
adopted at intervals ; and in a fhort time
he recovered the natural excretion of his
bowels, and in lefs than fix weeks after his
reafon and the ufe of his limbs, fo as to
be able to attend to his bufinefs as ufual.

C A S E   XCVII.

IN May 1795, I vifited Mr. A. H. rather
tall in ftature, of an atrabilarious complexion, about thirty-eight years of age,
who for feveral years paft had been fubject to an *exudatio pone aures,* which had
appeared periodically every fpring and
fall for feveral years, and generally
continued for the fpace of fix or eight
weeks; but the fpring was now far advanced without the leaft fign of its ufual
concomitant, and for fome time before
I faw him he had been inattentive to his
ufual

uſual concerns, and was ſunk into a habit
of anxiety, vexation, and diſguſt; was ſuſpicious, harſh, and laconic; captious, and
inquiſitive about trifles; extremely irritable, particularly at meals, and conceived
an inveterate averſion againſt a near relation who had never offended him, but on
the contrary, ſhewn him many marks of
diſintereſted friendſhip and regard. Having in his moments of dejection attempted
ſelf-violence, a perſon was provided to
attend him, and coercion had been found
neceſſary; but no recourſe had been had
to medical aſſiſtance of any kind. His
ſleep was little and interrupted, he had
frequent fluſhings in his face, and the
aſpect peculiar to inſane perſons; he always
looked aſkance at any one who came
near him, and in converſation was perpetually ſhifting his ideas from one ſubject
to another. The belly was conſtipated;
he had a full, hard, but rather ſlow pulſe;
the tongue was hard, ſkin dry and hot,
and his taſte impaired. He was very ſubject to eructation, and ſometimes diſcharg-
ed by retching a ſharp acrid matter.

I directed

I directed twelve ounces of blood to be taken from the arm, which, when cold, was covered with a yellow cruft, and afforded but little ferum. On the following day an emetic, confifting of two grains of antimonium tartarifatum, and one ounce of vinum ipecacuanha, was given, which brought away a great quantity of dark-coloured bile; the kali tartar. was next adminiftered in the quantity of fix drachms in barley-water, and a blifter was applied to the back, and kept open for more than a fortnight; but this producing no good effect, was then dried up, and foon afterwards fucceeded by a feton paffed between the fhoulders in the direction of the fpine, that difcharged very copioufly; and cooling aperients being given occafionally, the maniacal appearances gradually receded, and the patient in a few weeks becoming quiet and governable, and recovering his former fenfes, his attendant was only continued with him as a companion for fome time, and then totally difmiffed. An

iffue

iffue having been previoufly opened in his arm, the feton was fuffered to heal up; and although the ufual exudation from behind the ears has not fince returned, yet by the fubftituted difcharge from the iffue, proper refpect to diet, and faline laxatives when requifite, he has completely reco-vered his intellectual and bodily health.

CASE XCVIII.

ON the twenty-fecond of September 1795, I was fent for to a lady in the vici-nity of Stepney, who had a few weeks before been feized with a rotatory verti-go, attended with diminution of fight, and inability to ftand. Soon after the parox-yfm fhe was bled, and afterwards cupped with fcarifications, then bliftered, and an emetic was given. The caufe was attri-buted to hyfteria, owing to irregular and defective menftruation. Unufual and un-provoked anger, laughter, unremitting
vociferation,

vociferation, and diforderly inconfiftence of ideas fupervening, the cafe became manifeftly maniacal.

When I vifited her fhe appeared fad and thoughtful, and reluctantly anfwered to any queftion I propofed; and when fhe did fpeak, it was with a quick and fudden agitation. Her eyes rolled, and the face was convulfed. She was fubject to hyfteric ftrangulation, fpafmodic panting, flufhing of the face, and four eructation, and had phlogiftical blotches on feveral parts of her body. After an emetic, opium combined with the fœtid gums and fteel, were prefcribed. To remove the fpafmodic conftriction, the vapour-bath was recommended and ufed, as well as manu and pediluvium, upon the principles of revulfion, and a feton was opened *inter fcapulas* in the direction of the fpine; and by a ftrict perfeverance in a neceffary courfe of diet, under the unremitting care and moft excellent management of a confidential fervant, fhe gradually recovered a perfect reftoration of health and reafon, and has continued well ever fince.

CASE

CASE XCIX.

IN July 1797, I was defired to vifit the wife of a tradefman in Leadenhall-Street, who had become infane in confequence of an unfortunate parturition. On in-quiry I found an eminent practitioner had been confulted, who had advifed bleeding and an emetic, directed the fteams of hot vinegar to be often inhaled, that warm fomentations fhould often be ufed to her hands and feet, and that a blifter fhould be applied to her back, and continued open for a confiderable time. It was more than a month after her delivery that I firft faw her, when her afpect fufficiently indicated the fituation of her mind. She laboured under confiderable delirium, with great anxiety of fpirits, was continu-ally changing her pofture, and very irri-table; her face feemed flufhed with heat, her eyes were prominent and wild, fhe was coftive, and her ftools were dry, hard, and covered with a dark bilious humour; her urine little and high-coloured; her

tafte

tafte and hearing were both much impaired, with a pepfia, hyfteric ftrangulation, and
vain efforts to vomit. She was very frequently fubject to an uncommon gurgling
of the bowels ; her eye-lids were puffed,
red, and inflamed ; fhe often complained
of feeing red images before her eyes; her
delirium often rofe to fury; and fhe had
an accumulation of blood, with hardnefs,
inflammation, and tenfion in the left
breaft, to which a fuppurating cataplafm
was immediately applied ; and as fhe had
often fruitlefs retchings to vomit, an emetic was exhibited, and repeated every other
evening fucceffively to the third time.
The hair was cut off, and the crown of
her head fhaved, which was fometimes
rubbed with a flefh brufh, previous to a
fomentation of acetated fpirits of wine
with camphor. A fuppuration of the
affected breaft gave vent to a confiderable
difcharge of coagulated blood and pus;
and the pulfe being in a ftate to bear the
operation, venefection was ordered, and
repeated as occafion required. Soluble tartar in barley-water was given at intervals,

as a cooling aperient, and a feton opened
between the fhoulders in the direction of
the fpine. The dietetic regimen was cool,
flender, and attenuating; and to mollify
the rigidity of the fibres, the warm bath
was propofed and ufed twice a-day; during which time a powder of equal parts
of fal martis, myrrh, and fugar, was given
three times a-day in a ftrong infufion of
horfe-radifh; and at the end of two
months the cafe terminated favourably,
attended with regular returns of her ufual
periods.

———

CASE C.

IN the fubfequent cafe, although the diforder was very vifible in his countenance,
the gentleman was at intervals capable of
tranfacting his bufinefs as an attorney,
with wonderful facility and precifion; yet
foon after it became abfolutely neceffary
to confine him. When in the moft furious
ftage of his diforder, his paffion was inftantly
softened

foftened and his turbulence affuaged by
the mufic of a guitar, to which at other
times he paid but little attention. And
this in many other inftances has frequently
occurred, even where the mind has been
depreffed and funk into the deepeft abyfs
of melancholy; as is evinced by many
paffages of Scripture, and well expreffed
by a very ingenious bard of modern celebrity, in the following lines:

" All-powerful harmony, that can affuage
" And calm the forrows of the frenzied wretch,
" Till lull'd by thy enchanting grateful numbers
" He throws quite off the burthen that opprefs'd him."

When I was confulted in his cafe, he complained very much of tenfion and hardnefs in the left hypochonder, for which I
ordered the abdominal fibres and mufcles
on that fide to be frequently rubbed with
olive oil ftrongly impregnated with camphor. The head was fhaved and bathed
with vinegar and camphor, and the
fhower-bath was ufed every night and
morning for the fpace of fix weeks; but
finding no good effect from this practice,
and as emetics and blifters had before been

repeat-

repeatedly tried without effect, cupping with fcarification was next thought of, to which fucceeded cathartics by way of revulfion, and finally a feton between the fhoulders; but all to no purpofe; he continued as much deranged as ever, and at length died of an hydro thorax. On ftrict inquiry I difcovered the remote caufe in an hereditary predifpofition to madnefs, brought into action in the earlier part of his life by difappointed love.

CASE CI.

WITH an hereditary difpofition to infanity, an amiable young lady in the twenty-third year of her age, from mifplaced affection, fuddenly became infane. In November 1797 I firft faw her, when fhe had loft all command over the evacuation of fæces and urine, prone to mifchief, and had loft all he ral delicacy of manners. Her difappo ment had taken deep poffeffion of her heart and foul;

foul; her voice was low, languid, flow, and faltering, and fhe articulated very indiftinctly; her face was pale and wan; her appetite for food was obliterated; fhe would often fetch deep involuntary fighs, or emit fcreams and ejaculations, and then laugh, fing, and talk alternately; her tongue and fkin were dry, her fleep was fhort and interrupted, her menftruation deficient and painful; her tafte, fmell, and hearing were impaired; fhe was fubject to borborygmi, with vain efforts to vomit; her eye-lids were tumid and red; fhe would often bite her nails to the quick, and invincibly refufe all kind of fuftenance, except tea or water, and thofe in the fmalleft quantities. In this deplorable extremity, her eyes deep funk in their fockets, her cheeks miferably contracted, her neck bent forward and bowed with wretchednefs; her looks expreffive of all that fettled gloom of melancholy, and that corroding care, ſuch confume with perpetual angui ſhe continued near a month after I had feen her, when the

blefling

bleffing of death relieved her from all
her miferies.

CASE CII.

A. W. a young man of the moft refpectable family and connections, on the offer
of his hand in marriage to a young lady
being rejected, his mind inftantly became
detached from every object of pleafure,
he was fufpicious, tormented with doubts
and jealoufies, reftlefs and eafily agitated
to the moft vehement paffion on the moft
trifling occafions; he ftudioufly avoided
all fociety, and the converfation of his
relations and friends, and at length was
reduced to the moft deplorable extreme
of melancholic madnefs, in which unhappy
ftate I found him in the month of June
1794, when he appeared abfent to every
external object, greatly emaciated, with
every appearance of general debility; and
being naturally of a weakly conftitution,
                                         and

and delicate frame, notwithftanding the united endeavours of myfelf and many other medical practitioners, he fell a victim to his ill-fated paffion, and died tabid in the twenty-feventh year of his age.

CASE CIII.

A GENTLEMAN in a military capacity, much efteemed by his acquaintance for the brilliancy of his underftanding and the affability of his manners, in the beginning of February 1798, became deeply fmitten with the charms of a young lady of fuperior fortune and ftation in life, who having rejected his addreffes with difdain, and foon after married to another, he became gloomy, penfive, and low-fpirited; fhunned fociety, neglected his drefs, and all the duties of his ftation. Infurmountable dejection foon after followed, which terminated in confirmed infanity. He had an uncommon gloominefs of countenance, and

and a falfe conception of the nature of his own fpecies, fancying himfelf fometimes one animal and fometimes another, haraffed by the corrofion of mental pain, and finking under the weight of defpondence, he had twice attempted to put an end to his exiftence, but both proving ineffectual, he was the more clofely watched and attended to.

By a near relation of his who applied to me, the cafe was very accurately ftated as above, and I was further informed that for fome time before the beginning of his prefent complaint, he had frequently been fubject to eruptions of the fcorbutic kind, for which, by the advice of a phyfician, he had an iffue in his arm that had been dried up; and as thofe eruptions had not re-appeared for a confiderable time, I was induced to direct a feton between the fhoulders, which foon after took place, combined with every medical affiftance that could be thought of; but I was difappointed in the hopes of relieving him, as he became more and more debilitated,

both

both in body and mind, and at length died in the phrenſy of deſpair.

Innumerable are the fatal inſtances of human reaſon, ſubjugated by the irreſiſtible power and force of ill-regulated and ill-requited love *, which in its more pure and tranquil ſtate, is the moſt propitious gift of heaven,

---

* This was peculiarly exemplified in the caſe of the late unfortunate Mr. William Thweed, who died at Hoxton in April laſt. He was a man of a moſt unblemiſhed charaƈter, and of a temper remarkably mild. In the early part of his life he became enamoured of a young lady, the daughter of a clergyman near Bedford, whom he loved with the warmeſt enthuſiaſm; but from ſome diſagreements in ſettling the preliminaries of their marriage between their parents, the match was broken off, and all further intercourſe between the lovers forbidden. A cruel mandate, that was borne by the lady with coldneſs and indifference. The coldneſs of one whom he ſo tenderly loved, and the diſappointment he experienced, when his hopes were in their zenith, had ſo powerful an effeƈt upon his ſpirits, that his intelleƈts became diſordered, and he was for ſeveral years, at intervals, in a ſtate of inſanity, which gaining upon him for the laſt ten years of his life, he became a melancholy inhabitant of the receptacle for lunatics, where he died.

The

The cordial drop that heav'n in our cup has thrown,
To make the bitter pill of life go down,

Yet when fo unfortunately circumftanced
as to deviate into the agonies of mental
pain and anxiety, into nervous languor
and habitual and hopelefs dejection of
fpirits, fo as to induce a difordered ftate of
the brain, it ceafes to be a blefling, and
becomes an evil, of which the following
fketch, from the pen of the immortal
Thomfon, exhibits a very beautiful pic-
ture :

But abfent, what fantaftic woes arous'd,
Rage in each thought, by reftlefs mufing fed,
Chill the warm cheek, and blaft the bloom of life!
Neglected fortune flies, and fliding fwift
Prone into ruin fall his fcorn'd affairs.
'Tis nought but gloom around, the darken'd fun
Lofes his light ; the rofy-bofom'd fpring
To weeping fancy pines ; and yon bright arch
Contracted bends into a dufky vault.
All nature fades, extinct, and fhe alone,
Heard, felt, and feen, poffeffes every thought,
Fills every fenfe, and pants in every vein.

CASE

C A S E CIV.

AMONG the various fpecies of mania, we find no one more fingularly curious than that wherein the patient knows, feels, and laments his own pitiable ftate of mind, of which I prefume there are few more ftriking inftances than thofe which follow. A few years ago, Mr. J. W. an eminent bookfeller in Fleet-Street, the fon of a celebrated divine and mathematician, whofe uncommon parts and more uncommon learning, were more than equalled by his fingular and very extraordinary character. The fon very liberally inherited his father's talents, nor was the flatus hypochondrifi without its fhare in his patrimony; and as he intenfely felt, and could defcribe and conceive the degradation of his underftanding as defcending from paternal effect, the appellation of *fenfible madnefs* may perhaps not improperly be allowed as a diftinction to this clafs of mania. He naturally poffeffed a tender texture of the nervous fyftem, which

which as he knew the influence of his diforder was fo powerful as to deftroy all
hopes of remedy, foon reduced him to
a habit of anxiety, vexation, and difguft; yet he could pretty regularly attend to the ordinary duties and cere-
monies of life; obey the ufual folicitations to the natural excretions, the
feafonable returns of reft and fleep, and
the other demands of cuftom, nature, and
decency, with due decorum and regularity; but at intervals he was low,
dejeƈted, and tormented and perplexed
with the moft diftreffing and melancholy
thoughts and ideas. Every medical aid
was adminiftered in vain; change of refidence and dietetic regimen afforded but
temporary relief, and there frequently was
fuch a ftruggle between his own natural
good fenfe, and the falfe fuggeftions he laboured under, as to make him exclaim in the
agonizing anxiety of his mental fufferings,
" That he poffeffed the *mens confcia reƈti,*
and yet was totally unhappy and uncom-
fortable in himfelf; that he knew the feeds
of that dreadful malady he inherited, to be
fo

fo deeply rooted in his conftitution, as not
to admit the moft forlorn hope of relief;
that in vain he turned away from the
world, and fought folitary feclufion, for
there he was in danger from his own
miferable feelings of being tempted to
felf-deftruction; that his circumftances he
knew by his own induftry to be eafy, and
even affluent; that he had an internal
conviction of a merciful and good Creator,
and that there was a ftate of future retri-
bution, and yet that he could not diveft
himfelf of the firm belief that he fhould
become the victim of eternal punifhment,
and that he was actually under the domi-
nion of evil invifible agents; that although
he knew of no harm he had ever done to
any one, yet it often involuntarily occurred to his mind, that there were people
who confpired againft his life, and who
only waited for a fit opportunity to murder him; that he knew his wife and family
to be good and amiable, devoted to his
intereft, and perfonally attached to him
by duty and inclination, and yet his mental inquietude was fuch that he could not
help

help entertaining the greateſt averſion to them, as well as to ſome particular perſons of his acquaintance, who had rendered him the kindeſt offices, and even beſtowed on him marks of the moſt diſintereſted kindneſs and friendſhip; and yet he could not help thinking thoſe very people meant to poiſon him, or had actually hired aſſaſſins to take away his life."

In this manner he frequently expreſſed himſelf, till at length the unremitting ſtruggles and diſeaſed feelings, excited by mental illuſion, obtained ſuch an entire aſcendancy over his reaſon, that every ray thereof became obliterated, and he degenerated into a ſettled melancholy, in which unhappy ſtate he laboured under every corporeal morbidity that can be conceived to attend it. His aſpect became ſordid and ſtupid, his eyes were ſunk deep in their ſockets, his cheeks were miſerably fallen in, his viſion and hearing became indiſtinct, and quite extenuated and exhauſted he died a victim to mental derangement and deſpair, in the fifty-third year of his age.

CASE

CASE CV.

IN the beginning of April 1799, Mr. C. W. a perfon of refpectability in the fervice of the navy, came and addreffed me in perfon with great gravity and compofure, on the cafe of a gentleman of his acquaintance, whom a *lunatic anceftry*, he faid, had at intervals expofed to the grievous attacks of mental perturbation and derangement. He very emphatically defcribed his friend as a man of good natural and acquired endowments, and of an open, gay, convivial difpofition, except when affected by nervous languor and dejection, from the fad thoughts of his hereditary misfortune, the impreffion of which produced an alloy to every enjoyment, and often induced a peevifh and petulant caft of temper; caufed him to neglect the duties of his profeffion, and frequently to fly from fociety: that his nerves were irritable, and eafily affected by the moft trifling occurrence; that he was unable to fupport himfelf independently
dently

dently of his own exertions, which often expofed him to the fevereft reflexions; that wine, by fteeping his fenfes in forgetfulnefs, had often given a temporary truce to his intellectual miferies ; but that after its effects went off, they recurred with aggravated pain and anguifh, and his torments became greater than ever, infomuch that life became a burthen, and fo infupportable as to make him wifh for its diffolution, and his mind became the feat of undefcribable pain and remorfe; and in thofe moments the fear of being obferved made him try to the utmoft of his power to hide the tempefts of his foul in privacy and retirement, which was no fooner done, than his mind, exquifitely alive to the fenfe of his unhappy ftate, hurried him back to his former fcenes of employment, and convinced him that peace and happinefs were no where within his reach : that books afforded him no relief, as he could not pay a proper attention to the fubject he was reading ; and after paffing over a few pages, his mind reverted to its former laffitude and difcontent; that he

was

was particularly diftreffed by the *sympa-thies* of his friends, more than by any other circumftance whatever, and could not refift the propenfity of affronting them, when through courtefy or commi-feration they offered him either advice or affiftance, though at the fame time he knew it proceeded from the pureft and moft difinterefted motives of pity and friendfhip; that he was at times fo fearful of meeting a human being, that he has been often known to fhut himfelf up for hours, and even nights and days, to hide the anguifh of his internal forrows : and that his antipathy to mankind increafes to fuch a degree, that without any thing naturally rancorous in his mind and dif-pofition, or indeed the leaft habitual ha-tred to his own fpecies, except what was imperioufly impofed by his difeafed per-ception, he fancies himfelf in great dan-ger of becoming a complete mifanthro-pift; in fhort, added he, the alarming progrefs of his conftitutional malady is fuch, and he fo fenfibly feels the progref-fively melancholy depredation of his own

under-

underſtanding, that there is not a wiſh of
his heart that affords him half the ſolace as
that of the privation of life, ſince he feels
himſelf ſo totally loſt to every reliſh of the
world, and its enjoyment."

Having finiſhed this recital, he delivered
to me a written paper, containing the ſub-
ſtance of the foregoing narrative, burſt into
tears, wrung his hands, and acknowledged
himſelf to be the unhappy patient whoſe
ſtate of mind he had ſo affectingly de-
ſcribed. Aſtoniſhed at this diſcloſure, I
endeavoured to infuſe the belief that
his caſe admitted of cure, at leaſt of
ſome certain palliation from medical
aſſiſtance; that his anxiety, languor,
and deſpondency, were more the effects
of weak and relaxed nerves, the tender
texture of which had been wounded by
his own diſeaſed imagination, than of that
inherent intellectual affection, which had
too powerfully forced itſelf upon his
mind, as the cauſe of his wounded and
afflicted ſpirit. This, though a mere co-
louring, appeared to have afforded ſome
returning hope to the heart of this truly
unfortunate man, whom I diſmiſſed with
the

the ftrongeft injunctions to comply with
fuch advice and prefcriptions as I had given
him, and with confidence to look forward
to the fpeedy removal of his mental fufferings, and the perfect enjoyment of health of
body and peace of mind. But by a letter
received in December laft, I found it
impoffible to eradicate the thorn which
rankled in his heart, the intellectual poifon being of too virulent and corrofive a
nature to be mitigated either by advice
or medicine; and much praife is due to the
timely interpofition of his friends, which
has fince prevented the unhappy inheritor
of this dreadful calamity from becoming
a victim on the altar of felf-deftruction.

The learned and excellent author of
Solitude, whom I have before quoted,
fpeaking of the mind labouring under the
grievous preffure of melancholy and dejection, judicioufly obferves, that the
fecrecy and filence with which perfons of
this defcription ufually conceal the pangs
that torture their minds, is among the
moft dangerous fymptoms of the difeafe.
It is not, indeed, eafy to hide from the

anxious

anxious and penetrating eye of real friendfhip the feelings of the heart; but to the
carelefs and indifferent multitude of common acquaintances, the countenance may
wear the appearance not only of compofure, but even of gaiety, while the foul
is inwardly fuffering the keeneft anguifh
of unutterable woe; and as a cafe in point,
gives the following curious anecdote.

The celebrated Carlini, a French actor
of great merit, and in high reputation
with the public for the life, whim, frolic,
and vivacity with which he nightly entertained the Parifian audiences, applied to
a phyfician to whom he was not perfonally known, for advice, and reprefented
to him, that he was fubject to attacks of
the deepeft melancholy. The phyfician
advifed him to amufe himfelf by fcenes of
pleafure, and particularly directed him to
frequent the Italian comedy, "for," faid
he, "your diftemper muft be rooted indeed, if the acting of the *lively Carlini* does
not remove it." "Alas!" exclaimed the
unhappy patient, "I am the *very Carlini*
whom you recommend me to fee; and
while

while I am capable of filling Paris with mirth and laughter, I am myſelf the de-jected victim of melancholy and chagrin."

IN a power of fuch efficacy as medical electricity, fo well known to increafe fenfible perfpiration, accelerate the circulation of the blood, and promote the glandular fecretions, it is no wonder we are furnifhed from different authors with fuch a variety of well-attefted cafes, in which it has been ufed with confiderable advantage and fuccefs. In feveral cafes of St. Vitus's dance, and other fpafmodic affections of recent ftanding, in eruptions of the head and face, ophthalmia, deafnefs, hoarfenefs,*_lofs of fpeech_, chlorofis, defective or obftructed catamenia, even of the moft obftinate nature, I have adminiftered permanent benefit from electric friction, the fparks, fhocks, or fluid. The ufe of them in many fpecies of mania, I never found did the leaft harm; and although it muft be confeffed that in by far the greater number

---

* Vide, entire Recovery of Speech by Electricity, publifhed in the fourth volume of Memoirs of the Medical Society, in a cafe communicated by the Author the 25th of March 1793.

of cafes, electricity has afforded but a
partial or temporary relief at beft, yet in
the three following inftances it muft be
allowed to have effected a total cure.

_____

CASE CVI.

Mrs. E. W. was reduced to a miferable
ftate of melancholy from the death of her
hufband: fhe had for many months tried
every method of cure without effect. On
the 11th of March 1792, fhe was committed to my care and management, without any very fanguine hope of relief.
As electricity was the only probable
means left untried, foon after her admiffion I began with it in the moft fimple
form; proceeded next to electric friction,
and after a few days paffed fome electric
fhocks through the cranium, which I continued once in a day for nearly a month,
when fhe appeared confiderably better in
every refpect, and was capable of dreffing
and undreffing herfelf, and began to feed
herfelf,

herself, which she had not done before for many weeks prior to her being sent from home. The shocks were gradually increased every second, third, or fourth day, but not altogether confined to the head, for a month longer ; soon after which she was taken home by a near relation, and has since had no return of her disorder.

CASE CVII.

MR. T. H. a young gentleman, had long been in a low kind of delirium without a fever, with a constant anxiety of mind, without any apparent cause frequently shedding tears, yet unable to assign any reason, with tremblings, paleness of the countenance, extenuation of the body, and most other symptoms of confirmed melancholy. He was naturally of a hypochondriac cast, and predisposed to melancholy. The affections of his mind had been much increased by terrible watch-

watchfulnefs, fcarcely being able to obtain an hour's fleep for eight-and-forty hours together. He had been bliftered, cupped with and without fcarification, ufed both the cold and warm bath, taken purges, antimonial emetics, been bled, had a feton between the fhoulders, taken opium, bark, fteel, joined with aromatics; and to ufe the words of his father, had *"been drenched and fteeped to the chin in medicine, to no fort of purpofe."*

He was placed with me the latter end of September 1794, when having no chance left but electricity, I had immediate recourfe thereto, by applying the electric friction to his head, his body, and extremities, daily for the fpace of three weeks; at the end of which he became tolerably converfant, and could affift himfelf in the natural demands of nature, which he had been unable to do for a confiderable time paft; he got more fleep than ufual, and was obferved to perfpire when in bed, efpecially towards morning. Encouraged by this alteration for the better, I advanced in my procefs, and proceeded to

pafs

pafs gentle fhocks through the head, previoufly covered with flannel. Thefe were
gradually increafed till his fpirits became
uniform; he could walk about by himfelf,
find amufement in reading and writing,
and decently acquit himfelf at table with
the family. In lefs than three months
his anxiety and diftrefs of mind were entirely obliterated, and on returning home
foon after Chriftmas, by feeking agreeable
company, various recreations, and frequent change of refidence, and entirely
relinquifhing that intenfe application to
ftudy, and fedentary kind of life to which
he had been too much habituated before
his illnefs, has had no return of his
complaint.

CASE CVIII.

M<small>RS. S.</small> foon after a painful parturition of twins, who died foon after their
birth, became greatly troubled with the
milk fever, which, by the means of diaphoretics,

retics, gentle evacuations, and proper top i-
cal applications, terminated in a few days
after its commencement; but foon afterwards fhe was obferved to be very different in her actions and behaviour to what
fhe had been before her lying-in, and
betrayed ftrong fymptoms of mental derangement, which gradually increafed to
confirmed melancholy, with all its horrid
train of fears, forrows, and defpondencies.
She had a diftafte and diflike to every
thing, frequently not fpeaking a word in
a whole night and day together, never
taking the ufual notice of either her hufband or children, nor paying the leaft attention to her houfehold concerns. Great
laffitude, lofs of ftrength, and obftinate coftivenefs followed, for which the ufual laxatives were given, and the beft medical advice adminiftered; but getting no better,
early in May laft fhe was fent to my houfe.
The foluble tartar was given to relieve
her coftivenefs, and electricity occurring to
me as the moft likely effective means to
be of fervice to her, in a few days after
her admiffion, I began with fimple electri-
fication,

fication, and proceeded next to electric friction of the head and body, which having
continued daily for near a month, without
perceiving any change for the better, I determined to apply the ball of a glaſs-mounted
director connected to the conductor by a
wire to the region of the navel, and pouring a ſtream of electric ſparks into the abdomen, extracted them by a ball applied up
and down the ſpine: this being unremittingly continued for more than a month
longer, produced every good effect that
could be expected from returning reaſon
and habitual menſtruation *.

* Amongſt ſeveral extraordinary cures performed by
Mr. John Birch, ſurgeon, and publiſhed in 1792, in a
letter to the late ingenious mechanic Mr. George Adams,
on the ſubject of medical electricity, we find three caſes
of *melancholy*, two of which were entirely cured by the
ſole influence of electric application.

F I N I S.

SOME few cafes of puerperal fever, attended with fubfequent mania, *that have been tranfmitted to the London Medical Society, which after being read and ordered to be added to their manufcripts, might fufficiently have fanctioned their appearance in the prefent collection; but as fuch an addition muft necefarily have too much fwelled the fize of this volume, the Author has referved thofe communications for future publication.*

London: printed by R. NOBLE,
in the Old Bailey.

Classics in Psychiatry

An Arno Press Collection

Feuchtersleben, Ernst [Freiherr] von. **The Principles Of Medical Psychology.** 1847

Georget, [Etienne-Jean]. **De La Folie:** Considérations Sur Cette Maladie. 1820

Haslam, John. **Observations On Madness And Melancholy.** 1809

Hill, Robert Gardiner. **Total Abolition Of Personal Restraint In The Treatment Of The Insane.** 1839

Janet, Pierre [Marie-Felix] and F. Raymond. **Les Obsessions Et La Psychasthénie.** 1903. Two volumes

Janet, Pierre [Marie-Felix]. **Psychological Healing.** 1925. Two volumes

Kempf, Edward J. Psychopathology. 1920

Kraepelin, Emil. **Manic-Depressive Insanity And Paranoia.** 1921

Kraepelin, Emil. **Psychiatrie:** Ein Lehrbuch Für Studirende Und Aerzte. 1896

Laycock, Thomas. **Mind And Brain.** 1860. Two volumes in one

Liébeault, A[mbroise]-A[uguste]. **Le Sommeil Provoqué Et Les États Analogues.** 1889

Mandeville, B[ernard] De. **A Treatise Of The Hypochondriack And Hysterick Passions.** 1711

Morel, B[enedict] A[ugustin]. Traité Des Degénérescences Physiques, Intellectuelles Et Morales De L'Espèce Humaine. 1857. Two volumes in one

Morison, Alexander. **The Physiognomy Of Mental Diseases.** 1843

Myerson, Abraham. **The Inheritance Of Mental Diseases.** 1925

Perfect, William. **Annals Of Insanity.** [1808]

Pinel, Ph[ilippe]. **Traité Médico-Philosophique Sur L'Aliénation Mentale.** 1809

Prince, Morton, et al. Psychotherapeutics. 1910

Psychiatry In Russia And Spain. 1975

Ray, I[saac]. **A Treatise On The Medical Jurisprudence Of Insanity.** 1871

Semelaigne, René. **Philippe Pinel Et Son Oeuvre Au Point De Vue De La Médecine Mentale.** 1888

Thurnam, John. **Observations And Essays On The Statistics Of Insanity.** 1845

Trotter, Thomas. **A View Of The Nervous Temperament.** 1807

Tuke, D[aniel] Hack, editor. **A Dictionary Of Psychological Medicine.** 1892. Two volumes

Wier, Jean. **Histoires, Disputes Et Discours Des Illusions Et Impostures Des Diables, Des Magiciens Infames, Sorcieres Et Empoisonneurs.** 1885. Two volumes

Winslow, Forbes. **On Obscure Diseases Of The Brain And Disorders Of The Mind.** 1860

Burdett, Henry C. **Hospitals And Asylums Of The World.** 1891-93. Five volumes. 2,740 pages on NMA standard 24x-98 page microfiche only